Recovery-Stress
Questionnaire for Athletes:
User Manual

Recovery-Stress Questionnaire for Athletes: User Manual

Michael Kellmann, PhD
University of Potsdam

K. Wolfgang Kallus, PhD
University of Graz

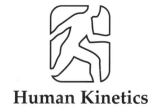

Human Kinetics

Library of Congress Cataloging-in-Publication Data

Kellmann, Michael, 1965-
[Erholungs-Belastungs-Fragebogen für Sportler. English]
The recovery-stress questionnaire for athletes : user manual / Michael Kellmann, K.
Wolfgang Kallus.
p. cm.
Includes bibliographical references.
ISBN 0-7360-3776-4 (manual) -- ISBN 0-7360-4087-0 (software)
1. Sports--Psychological aspects--Handbooks, manuals, etc. 2. Stress
(Psychology)--Testing--Handbooks, manuals, etc. 3. Stress
(Physiology)--Testing--Handbooks, manuals, etc. 4. Athletes--Psychological
testing--Handbooks, manuals, etc. I. Kallus, K. Wolfgang (Konrad Wolfgang) II. Title.

GV706.4 .K44 2001
796'.01--dc21
2001016807

ISBN: 0-7360-3776-4 (manual)
ISBN: 0-7360-4087-0 (software)

Acquisitions Editor: Michael S. Bahrke, PhD
Developmental Editor: Melissa Feld
Assistant Editors: Susan C. Hagan, Kim Thoren, and John Wentworth
Copyeditor: Barb Field
Proofreader: Sue Fetters
Permissions Managers: Courtney Astle and Dalene Reeder
Graphic Designer: Nancy Rasmus
Graphic Artist: Angela K. Snyder
Cover Designer: Keith Blomberg
Illustrator: Craig Newsom
Printer: Versa Press

Printed in the United States of America

10   9   8   7   6   5   4   3   2   1

Human Kinetics
Website: www.humankinetics.com

United States: Human Kinetics
P.O. Box 5076
Champaign, IL 61825-5076
800-747-4457
e-mail: humank@hkusa.com

Canada: Human Kinetics
475 Devonshire Road Unit 100
Windsor, ON N8Y 2L5
800-465-7301 (in Canada only)
e-mail: orders@hkcanada.com

Europe: Human Kinetics
Units C2/C3 Wira Business Park
West Park Ring Road
Leeds LS16 6EB, United Kingdom
+44 (0) 113 278 1708
email: hk@hkeurope.com

Australia: Human Kinetics
57A Price Avenue
Lower Mitcham, South Australia 5062
08 8277 1555
e-mail: liahka@senet.com.au

New Zealand: Human Kinetics
P.O. Box 105-231, Auckland Central
09-523-3462
e-mail: hkp@ihug.co.nz

Dedicated to all athletes and coaches
who participated in the development of the
Recovery-Stress Questionnaire for Athletes.

Contents

Information for the User of the Recovery-Stress Questionnaire for Athletes

Dear User,

Purchase of the Recovery-Stress Questionnaire for Athletes (RESTQ-Sport) manual includes the unusual option of photocopying as many copies of the questionnaire as you wish for applied or scientific purposes. The only requirement is that you purchase an original manual from Human Kinetics.

In the back of the manual you will find the Recovery-Stress Questionnaire for Athletes with 76 and 52 items, respectively, as well as the item listing and the scoring key. In case data assessment takes place in situations where no computer scoring is possible (e.g., on the track, in the gym, on the road), this package includes the hand scoring sheets for both questionnaires and an empty hand scoring profile sheet. However, it is more convenient to use the database program RESTQ-Sport for an easy calculation of the recovery-stress state. Brief instructions for the database program RESTQ-Sport can also be found in appendix B.

If you use the RESTQ-Sport in studies or in applied settings, the authors would like to receive feedback on your experience in working with this instrument. For the further development of the RESTQ-Sport, we ask that you send us a copy of the original data set, a sample description, and information about the study or intervention approach used.

If you have further questions or comments, please contact:

Dr. Michael Kellmann
University of Potsdam
Institute of Sport Science
Am Neuen Palais 10
14469 Potsdam
Germany
email: **kellmann@rz.uni-potsdam.de**
www.uni-potsdam.de/u/sportpsych/indexe.htm

If you purchase the RESTQ-Sport, you may use it as a research or monitoring tool for athletes during the training process. Athletes and coaches can modify the personal and training environment to optimize the training process and actively reduce the risk of overtraining. However, you should not use the RESTQ-Sport for selection purposes! Although the tendency for the results of psychological assessments to enter into selection decisions cannot be totally avoided, the practice is unethical and may destroy the trusting relationship between coach and athlete. Furthermore, if a serious, long-lasting unhealthy recovery-stress state is detected, consultation with a trained psychologist or counseling center is highly recommended.

Acknowledgments

Large projects such as the Recovery-Stress Questionnaire for Athletes (RESTQ-Sport) can only be realized through the unremitting efforts of creative and motivated people. Our special thanks to Wilhelm Janke for providing groundwork and assistance during the initial studies of the RESTQ-Sport. The concept and its development are closely tied to his biopsychological research and his study group on the themes of stress, coping, and emotion. We are grateful to Hans Eberspächer and Hans-Dieter Hermann for establishing the recovery-stress model in high performance sport. The RESTQ-Sport was originated, as well as validated from the medical viewpoint, in cooperation with Jürgen Steinacker, Werner Lormes, Uwe Gastmann, and Manfred Lehmann. As a result, the spectrum of the instrument has been broadened by its valuable potential for enlightening the psychological and physical factors of overtraining.

The involvement of Volker Stark made it possible for us to include in the survey coaches and athletes of the Federal Sports Association of Baden-Württemberg, Germany. The rowing coach Klaus-Dietrich Günther introduced the RESTQ-Sport to the Junior National Team of the German Rowing Association in 1994. We thank all athletes and coaches, as well as head coach Dieter Altenburg, for their continuous cooperation with the Junior National Rowing Team. Our colleagues in the United States, Canada, and in other European countries supported us with their open-mindedness during the empirical work for the RESTQ-Sport. In particular, Craig Wrisberg (University of Tennessee, U.S.A.), Cal Botterill (University of Winnipeg, Canada), John Hogg (University of Alberta, Canada), and Yuri Hanin (Research Institute for Olympic Sports, Finland) not only shared our enthusiasm for our work, but also gave us important inputs and motivated us to speed up the development of the RESTQ-Sport.

Data processing, data input, and varying analyses for the development and validation of the RESTQ-Sport would not have been possible without the patience of our research assistants. Angelika Eweleit, Clare Wilson, and Kim Raisner collected in their empirical studies important data for establishing this method. Clare Wilson, Fahreen Rayani, Natalie Posthumus, and John Hogg reviewed the English translation. Their comments and suggestions helped us improve the quality and enhance the meaningfulness of the manuscript, as well as avoid translation errors. Kim Raisner contributed to the construction of the manual by compiling the tables.

Appreciation is also expressed to Mike Bahrke for continuous support and to Melissa Feld for her highly professional editorial work.

We are happy to introduce the Recovery-Stress Questionnaire for Athletes. Our sincere thanks to all who were involved in the development process.

Introduction

The Recovery-Stress Questionnaire for Athletes (RESTQ-Sport) is an instrument that systematically reveals the *recovery-stress states* of athletes. The recovery-stress state indicates the extent to which persons are physically and/or mentally stressed, whether or not they are capable of using individual strategies for recovery, as well as which strategies are used. The RESTQ-Sport is structured in modules. The basic RESTQ module by Kallus (1995) was not constructed for a specific field of application; rather, it was continuously developed through fundamental biopsychological research in the problem area of stress. The basic RESTQ module was later extended by seven sport-specific scales to assess the full complexities of stress and recovery in athletes.

The RESTQ-Sport was constructed by Kallus (1995) to obtain a differentiated answer to the question "How are you?" Initially, a primary objective in compiling the items was to look for ways to predict the stress reactions of individuals in their present state. Additionally, this idea centered on the everyday observation that individuals in need of a vacation obviously react differently to demands than individuals who currently have a high degree of psychological and physical fitness. In sport, the connection between the current recovery-stress situation and competition or training achievement is obvious (Kallus & Kellmann, 2000; Kellmann & Günther, 2000; Kellmann & Kallus, 1993). Also, in a training camp, where the extent and intensity of the training are deliberately increased, the subjective assessment is important because it can reveal insufficient recovery. This situation can result in performance decrease, overtraining, burnout, or dropping out of sports (e.g., see Budgett, 1998; Kallus & Kellmann, 2000; Kellmann & Günther, 2000; Lehmann, Foster, & Keul, 1993; Lehmann, Foster, Gastmann, Keizer, & Steinacker, 1999). These nega-

tive effects are also a risk in competitive programs that are too strenuous or too critical. As noted by Hollmann (1989) a decade ago, "in this way the athlete is rushed from one peak to the other and the recovery phases become too short in today's limits of human performance" (p. 79). For a conscious integration of recovery phases in the competition and training cycles, it is desirable to train athletes in close cooperation among coaches, sport physicians, and sport psychologists, thus utilizing the available medical, psychological, and performance data on an interdisciplinary basis.

The Recovery-Stress Questionnaire for Athletes reveals their current recovery-stress states and outlines a differentiated picture of the actual extent of stress that constitutes an athlete's stress state. The questionnaire is based on the hypothesis that an accumulation of stress in different areas of life, at least with insufficient recovery possibilities, leads to a changed psychophysical general state. As the initial state changes, the athlete's capacity to act and perform changes, along with their potential for adapting to further stressors (Kallus, 1992).

As a multidimensional questionnaire, the RESTQ-Sport is especially suitable for clarification of the interdependencies of stress and recovery activities. For this purpose, the questionnaire records the frequency of stress and recovery. Furthermore, it differentiates nonspecific and sport-specific areas of stress and recovery. By recording recovery and stress at the same time, the RESTQ-Sport closes a theoretically as well as practically important gap, illustrated by the review "Overtraining and Recovery" by Kenttä and Hassmén (1998). These authors characterize the RESTQ-Sport as one of the few questionnaires that "attempts to address the full complexities of stress and recovery" (p. 12).

PART I
Description and Application

CHAPTER 1

Description of the Recovery-Stress Questionnaire for Athletes

The Recovery-Stress Questionnaire for Athletes (RESTQ-Sport) was developed to measure the *frequency of current stress along with the frequency of recovery-associated activities*. The current recovery-stress state depends on preceding stress and recovery activities. Through the simultaneous assessment of stress and recovery, a differentiated picture of the current recovery-stress state can be provided. The specific characteristics of the RESTQ-Sport are that it allows systematic and direct measurement of appraised events, states, and activities regarding their frequency while simultaneously considering stress and recovery processes.

With 19 scales, the RESTQ-Sport assesses potentially stressful and restful events and their subjective consequences during *the past three days/nights*. Without essential changes in the internal consistency of the scales, the period of reference can be extended up to four weeks, depending on the research question (Kallus, 1995; Kallus & Kellmann, 2000). The appraisal of the recovery-stress state in the RESTQ is a result of a quantitative assessment of the frequency of stress and recovery activities in the past three days/nights. The questionnaire considers subjectively appraised events and states. Basing the method on the concepts of overload and stress is well founded in that there is a transactional relationship between conditions and actively appraising persons.

The Recovery-Stress Questionnaire for Athletes comprises 76 statements (items) plus an introductory item (warm-up item), which is not included in the scoring. Each scale of the RESTQ-76 Sport consists of four items (see appendix C). A shorter version (RESTQ-52 Sport) with 52 items is also available (see appendix D). Both forms refer to the past three days/nights.

Description of the Scales

The Recovery-Stress Questionnaire for Athletes is based on the basic module, RESTQ-48 (items of RESTQ-24A and RESTQ-24B), consisting of seven stress scales and five recovery scales (Kallus, 1995). Scales 1 through 7 consider life stresses in general (whether temporary or stable), performance-related stress, and physical aspects of stress, and scales 8 through 12 consider temporary or stable nonspecific recovery activities.

Seven sport-specific areas assess additional aspects of stress (scales 13 through 15) and recovery (scales 16 through 19). Table 1.1 provides an overview of the RESTQ-Sport scales.

General Stress covers nonspecific stress reactions that manifest themselves in frequent indications of mental stress, depressed mood, and listlessness. This scale was labeled *General Stress* because of its consistently high correlation with the remaining stress scales (Kallus, 1995). *Emotional Stress* predominantly deals with anxiety, inhibitions, and irritation in the past few days. *Social Stress* measures the frequency of arguments, fights, irritation concerning others, and general upset. *Conflicts/Pressure* assesses whether conflicts were unresolved, unpleasant things had to be done, goals could not be reached, or certain thoughts could not be dismissed. *Fatigue* deals with being constantly disturbed during important work, as well as with overfatigue. A *Lack of Energy* indicates ineffective work behavior, such as a lack of concentration, energy, and decision making. *Physical Complaints* measured by the last stress-oriented scale relates to physical indisposition and complaints. *Success* relates to pleasure at work, having lots of ideas, and achievement. It is the only recovery-oriented scale that is concerned with

Table 1.1 Scales of the Recovery-Stress Questionnaire for Athletes

Scale	Scale Summary
1	**General Stress** Subjects with high values describe themselves as being frequently mentally stressed, depressed, unbalanced, and listless.
2	**Emotional Stress** Subjects with high values experience frequent irritation, aggression, anxiety, and inhibition.
3	**Social Stress** High values match subjects with frequent arguments, fights, irritation concerning others, general upset, and lack of humor.
4	**Conflicts/Pressure** High values are reached if in the preceding few days conflicts were unsettled, unpleasant things had to be done, goals could not be reached, and certain thoughts could not be dismissed.
5	**Fatigue** Time pressure in job, training, school, and life, being constantly disturbed during important work, overfatigue, and lack of sleep characterize this area of stress.
6	**Lack of Energy** This scale matches ineffective work behavior like inablity to concentrate and lack of energy and decision making.
7	**Physical Complaints** Physical indisposition and physical complaints related to the whole body are characterized by this scale.
8	**Success** Success, pleasure at work, and creativity during the past few days are assessed in this area.
9	**Social Recovery** High values are shown by athletes who have frequent pleasurable social contacts and change combined with relaxation and amusement.
10	**Physical Recovery** Physical recovery, physical well-being, and fitness are characterized in this area.
11	**General Well-Being** Besides frequent good moods and high well-being, general relaxation and contentment are also in this scale.
12	**Sleep Quality** Enough recovering sleep, an absence of sleeping disorders while falling asleep, and sleeping through the night characterize recovery sleep.

Scale	Scale Summary
13	**Disturbed Breaks** This scale deals with recovery deficits, interrupted recovery, and situational aspects that get in the way during periods of rest (e.g., teammates, coaches).
14	**Burnout/Emotional Exhaustion** High scores are shown by athletes who feel burned out and want to quit their sport.
15	**Fitness/Injury** High scores signal an acute injury or vulnerability to injuries.
16	**Fitness/Being in Shape** Athletes with high scores describe themselves as fit, physcially efficient, and vital.
17	**Burnout/Personal Accomplishment** High scores are reached by athletes who feel integrated in their team, communicate well with their teammates, and enjoy their sport.
18	**Self-Efficacy** This scale is characterized by how convinced the athlete is that he/she has trained well and is optimally prepared.
19	**Self-Regulation** The use of mental skills for athletes to prepare, push, motivate, and set goals for themselves are assessed by this scale.

performance in general. *Social Recovery* assesses the frequency of pleasurable social contacts and change combined with relaxation and amusement. *Physical Recovery* covers physiological relaxation and fitness. Besides the frequency of good mood and high well-being, general relaxation and being content are assessed by the *General Well-Being* scale. *Sleep Quality*, the final scale of the general Recovery-Stress Questionnaire, indicates absence of trouble falling asleep and interrupted sleep (Kallus, 1995).

The sport-specific scale *Disturbed Breaks* is sensitive to deficiencies of recovery and interrupted recovery during periods of rest (e.g., halftimes, timeouts), both of which can impair subsequent performance (Kellmann & Kallus, 1994). *Emotional Exhaustion* is characterized by wanting to give up or lack of persistence. This relates to any disappointments in the context of sport that might lead to quitting the sport. *Injury* consists of any statements dealing with injuries, vulnerability to injuries, and an impairment of physical strength. *Being in Shape* assesses subjective feelings about performance ability and competence, one's perceived fitness, and vitality. *Personal Accomplishment* primarily asks about appreciation and empathy within the team and the realization of personal goals in sport. *Self-Efficacy*

measures the level of expectation and competence regarding an optimal performance preparation in practice. *Self-Regulation* refers to the use of psychological skills training when preparing for performance (e.g., goal setting, mental training, motivation).

Temporal Stability of the Current Recovery-Stress State

The Recovery-Stress Questionnaire for Athletes endeavors to represent the recovery-stress state in temporary states, including physical, emotional, and behavioral aspects, with a certain persistence (Bradburn, 1969). Therefore, the recovery-stress state, in contrast to the actual condition, is stable in the face of temporary functional fluctuations.

The scores obtained should be considered independent of temporary and negligible conditional changes of state by means of a representation in the degree of stress and the extent of recovery in the past three days/nights. In addition, items were used that relate closely to behavior. Consequently, the scales show a high short-term stability, at least in the region of one to two days. Simultaneously, the RESTQ-Sport is conceived as an instrument that allows for the sensitive assessment of changes in a person's recovery-stress state and clearly monitors changes in stress and recovery, respectively.

The Recovery-Stress Questionnaire for Athletes and Related Instruments

The Recovery-Stress Questionnaire for Athletes represents an important addition to existing questionnaires that measure the occurrence of recent stress (Stone & Neale, 1984), the extent of subjective stress (Weyer & Hodapp, 1975), and the frequency of stressful daily hassles (Kanner, Coyne, Schaefer, & Lazarus, 1981). The RESTQ-Sport allows a person's present *condition of subjective stress* to be systematically and directly recorded in the form of a differentiated recovery-stress state. A special feature of the RESTQ is to record appraised events, conditions, and activities with regard to their frequency, capturing the recovery and stress processes simultaneously.

Until now, sport psychology research has dealt with the relationship between overtraining and emotional state and disposition. Research on emotional state is mostly based on the Profile of Mood States (POMS) (McNair, Lorr, & Droppleman, 1971, 1992), a self-rating instrument for the assessment of mood (*Tension, Depression, Anger, Vigor, Fatigue, Confusion*). For example, Morgan and colleagues (1987) reported mood changes in swimmers during the season. Early in the season, swimmers displayed the *iceberg profile* (Morgan, 1985; Morgan & Costill, 1996), a profile indicative of positive mental health that is associated with successful athletic performance. During overtraining, mood disturbances significantly increased and were accompanied by a profile reflecting diminished mental health. After the training intensity was significantly reduced, the swimmers again exhibited the original iceberg profile. More recently, the existence of a *dose-response relationship* was demonstrated between training volume and mood disturbances (Raglin, 1993). Increases in training volume parallel corresponding elevations in mood disturbance (e.g., more anger, depression, tension, fatigue, and less vigor and well-being). Mood improvements occur if training volume is reduced (Berger et al., 1999; Martin, Andersen, & Gates, 2000; Morgan, Brown, Raglin, O'Conner & Ellickson, 1987; Morgan, Costill, Flynn, Raglin, & O'Conner, 1988). Morgan and colleagues (1987) recommend that the symptoms associated with overtraining and staleness should be monitored continuously during the course of athletic training, so that training volumes can be adjusted as soon as negative symptoms begin to appear.

Since recovery can be characterized not merely as lack of stress (Kallus, 1995), but also as a proactive individualized process to reestablish psychological and physiological resources (Kellmann, in press), the POMS, which is the most frequently used measure, may be insufficient to explore recovery processes. The POMS was initially developed as an economical method of identifying and assessing transient, fluctuating affective states (McNair et al., 1992). Consequently, the POMS only vaguely reflects recovery processes. A more detailed assessment of these processes is needed for systematic development of training plans that combine intensive training and recovery in the form of dynamic, intensive processes.

The RESTQ-Sport assesses mood-oriented stress- and recovery-associated activities using items such as *I was angry with someone* or *I had a good time with my friends*. In other words, the RESTQ-Sport basically asks the question, "What happened in the past three days/nights?" and provides a differentiated picture of the current recovery-stress state based on 12 nonspecific and 7 additional sport-specific scales. This demonstrates how it differs from the POMS instrument, which only assesses the current mood state and therefore shows no specific starting points for intervention.

The evaluation based on the RESTQ-Sport scales and, in specific cases, also on the item level provides information about activities where "room for improvement" is obvious. This information can be used as an active component to modify behavior in the future. Consequently, since the consultant gets a clear picture of what happened during the preceding days for groups and/or individuals, the RESTQ-Sport is favorable in applied settings. Through the assessment of mood-oriented activities, the results of the RESTQ-Sport reflect a precise situational description of individual and/or group processes (Kellmann, Kallus, Günther, Lormes, & Steinacker, 1997). In addition, general and/or sport-specific activities can also be considered a cause and a mediator for mood states, which is supported by the considerable correlations between the RESTQ-Sport and the POMS (Kallus & Kellmann, 2000; Kellmann, 1999; Kellmann, Altenburg, Lormes, & Steinacker, 2001; Kellmann, Fritzenberg, & Beckmann, 2000; Kellmann & Günther, 2000; Kellmann & Kallus, 1999).

Summary

- The RESTQ-Sport assesses potentially stressful and restful events and their subjective consequences during *the past three days/nights*.

- The RESTQ-Sport provides a differentiated picture of the current *recovery-stress state* based on 12 nonspecific and 7 additional sport-specific scales.

- The current recovery-stress state, in contrast to the actual condition, is stable in the face of temporary functional fluctuations.

- Since recovery can be characterized not merely as lack of stress, but also as a proactive individualized process to reestablish psychological and physiological resources, the POMS may be insufficient to explore recovery processes.

- The RESTQ-Sport shows specific starting points for intervention.

CHAPTER 2

Application of the Recovery-Stress Questionnaire for Athletes

The Recovery-Stress Questionnaire for Athletes (RESTQ-Sport) can be applied in almost all settings: at team meetings, in classrooms, on the track, in the gym, or at the pool. This instrument is useful for all sports, and recently it was also found reliable and valid for German athletes with a physical handicap (Kellmann et al., 2000).

Instruction

The questionnaire is supplied with a cover sheet that gives detailed instructions on how to answer the questionnaire, including an example. In addition, the cover sheet contains the directive that the statements related to performance should refer to performance during competition, as well as during training or practice. This makes it possible to complete the questionnaire without the help of a third person. The cover sheet should be read thoroughly before starting the questionnaire.

Subjects are asked to fill out the RESTQ-Sport without taking any long breaks. While completing the questionnaire, subjects should be undisturbed, and it is important that each subject fill out the questionnaire individually. Depending on the ver-

sion, it takes between 8 and 12 minutes to answer the questionnaire the first time. After the test has been taken repeatedly, the completion time is reduced.

Item Format of the Recovery-Stress Questionnaire for Athletes

The Recovery-Stress Questionnaire for Athletes assesses potentially stressful events and their consequences, along with the frequency of recovery-associated activities and their effects in the past three days/nights. The items of the RESTQ-Sport identify activities or conditions in the form of *incomplete* sentences. Together with the time period given at the top of the page *(in the past (3) days/nights)*, each item forms a statement. A Likert-type scale is used with values ranging from 0 *(never)* to 6 *(always)* indicating how often the respondent participated in various activities during the *past three days/nights* (table 2.1). As with the general RESTQ, the sport-specific version includes a warm-up item that is not included in the analysis.

Table 2.1   Sample Item and Answer Mode of the RESTQ-Sport

In the past (3) days/nights

... I felt vulnerable to injuries

0	1	2	3	4	5	6
never	seldom	sometimes	often	more often	very often	always

Scoring

The scale values are calculated by taking the mean of the item values (checked numbers) (rounded off to two decimal points). The formation of the mean is appropriate because of the different number of questions in the various versions of the RESTQ-Sport. In case of missing data, the mean should only be calculated when at least 50% of the items of each scale have been answered. In the *Sleep Quality* scale, the items for disturbed sleep first have to be inverted (6 minus item value = rough item score; e.g., $6 \rightarrow 0; 5 \rightarrow 1; 4 \rightarrow 2; 3 = 3; 2 \rightarrow 4; 1 \rightarrow 5; 0 \rightarrow 6$). The scoring sheet in the appendix can be referred to for manual scoring. Additionally, the data can be represented graphically in a *recovery-stress state profile*.

The mean of each scale can range from 0 to 6. High scores in the stress-associated activity scales reflect intense subjective stress, whereas high scores in the recovery-oriented scales reflect plenty of recovery activities.

- The scales in the area of stress (scales 1-7) can be summarized in a general stress-oriented scale (mean of scales 1-7).

- Correspondingly, a total mean for recovery can be formed from the scales in a general recovery-related scale (scales 8-12).

- The same procedure applies for the sport-specific stress (mean of scales 13-15) and recovery areas (mean of scales 16-19).

- The general and sport-specific stress and recovery scales can be combined to calculate global overall stress and recovery scores, respectively. However, this procedure is only recommended for group comparisons.

Kallus (1995) stated that the covariance between the scales for recovery and stress is neither linear nor symmetrical. *Consequently, the calculation of one overall single score of all stress and recovery scales is strongly prohibited.*

Interpretation of Results

The RESTQ-Sport is constructed in accordance with the classical test theory (classical-latent-additive model; Moosbrugger, 1982). Therefore, an interpretation of the scale mean as an absolute value is not possible. Hence, the interpretation of the RESTQ-Sport profile should refer to either a reference group of the athlete, to intraindividual changes over time, or to the mean and variability of single samples found in the appendix. Moreover, it is important to check if the particular RESTQ-Sport version corresponds to the chosen reference period and the moment of testing of the respective comparison group.

The reference values in the appendix should not be misinterpreted as norms. The recovery-stress state varies during training camps, cycles of competitions, working weeks of a year, different phases of life, and as a result of specific stress and recovery activities. Therefore, the means in the appendix constitute a general situation-unspecific foundation and, as a result, should be interpreted as a *reference value* rather than as a norm.

Summary

- Depending on the version, the RESTQ-Sport can be completed in 8 to 12 minutes the first time. After the test has been taken repeatedly, the completion time is reduced.

- The items of the RESTQ-Sport identify activities or conditions in the form of *incomplete sentences*.

- The data can be represented graphically in a *recovery-stress state profile*.

- High scores in the stress-associated activity scales reflect intense subjective stress, whereas high scores in the recovery-oriented scales reflect plenty of recovery activities.

- The calculation of one overall single score of all stress and recovery scales is strongly prohibited.

- An interpretation of the scale mean as an absolute value is not possible. The interpretation of the RESTQ-Sport profile should be limited to a reference group of the user or to intraindividual changes over time.

CHAPTER 3

Individual-Specific Diagnostic Case Studies

The following cases are derived from Kallus and Kellmann (2000); Kellmann and Günther (1999); Kellmann, Kallus, Günther, et al. (1997); and Kellmann et al. (2001). On the first view the case studies look maybe simplistic but they should introduce some approaches the RESTQ-Sport can be utilized in applied settings. Each case study is divided into sections on description, diagnosis, and intervention. They illustrate the application of the RESTQ-Sport for diagnostic purposes and the subsequent intervention.

The main purpose is to identify athletes whose recovery-stress states during training camp do not correspond with the training schedule. Through early intervention, individual training can be adapted to help the athlete deal with training stress and prevent overtraining.

The internal consistencies for some scales bring about some limitations for individual diagnosis based on single scales. Therefore, the complete profile will be considered, and deviation on more than one scale will be used as a screening method for individual problems.

Three approaches can be applied for diagnostic purposes:

A. For individual assessment, an "area of tolerance" is calculated using the mean plus or minus the standard deviation (M ± 1 SD) of the whole team (see figure 3.1). If more than two scores deviate from this tolerance range, these athletes receive special attention. Since training volume changes throughout training camp (see chapter 6, figure 6.2), the area of tolerance must be recalculated for each measurement.

B. Individual profiles provide much detailed information about the changes in the recovery-stress state over time (see figures 3.2 and 3.3).

C. A combination of approaches A and B can also be applied.

In general, it should be noted that low scores in the stress-related areas and high scores in the recovery-related areas are "positively" labeled, and vice versa. However, in this context, terms such as *good/bad* or *positive/negative* do not exist. It must always be kept in mind that the RESTQ-Sport profile reflects just *one short period in a person's life*, which may change drastically within a few days.

Case 1: Rower A

Description and diagnosis: The first RESTQ-Sport assessment took place three days after the beginning of the training camp. Compared to the group, rower A seemed to be similarly stressed because her scores were in the area of tolerance (M ± 1 SD) except for on the *Fatigue* scale; however, her recovery-stress state revealed low scores in the *Physical Recovery* and *Sleep Quality* scales (figure 3.1). In combination with the *Fatigue* scale, it could be concluded that she was experiencing a lack of sleep.

Intervention: After consultation with the head coach, the coach of the boat contacted the rower and found a simple cause for her sleep deficit. She was sleeping in a bed that was in very bad shape, and she had trouble falling asleep at night and during the recovery times after lunch. After acquiring a board and putting it under the mattress, she slept better. Control measurements showed an improvement in *Physical Recovery*, a decrease in *Fatigue,* and clearly better scores in *Sleep Quality* despite a higher training load. The solution is not always that simple but is often easier than expected. In this case, the athlete did not talk to the coach at all about what bothered her but revealed the current situation in the RESTQ-Sport.

RESTQ-76 Sport Profile:

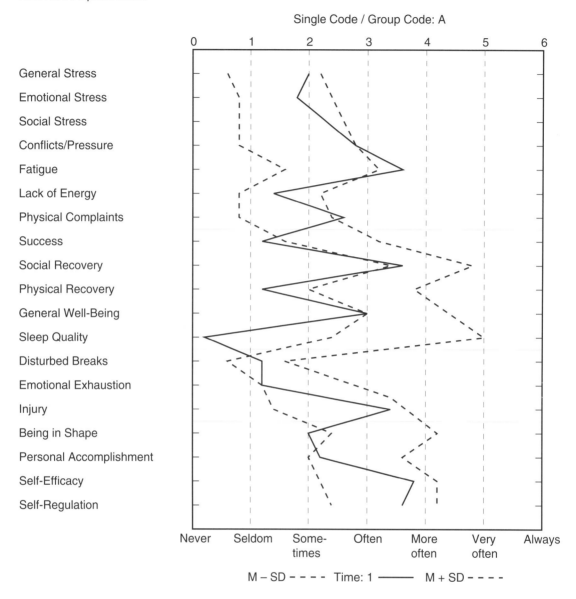

Figure 3.1 RESTQ-Sport profile for the female rower A and the area of tolerance for the total group (between the broken lines) for the first point of time in the survey (Trial: 1).

Adapted, by permission, from M. Kellmann and K.W. Kallus, 1999, Mood, Recovery-Stress State, and Regeneration. In *Overload, Fatigue, Performance Incompetence, and Regeneration in Sport*, edited by M. Lehmann et al. (New York: Plenum), 112.

Case 2: Rower B

Description: A 17-year-old athlete (rower B) became ill with an acute case of tonsillitis, which was medically treated. To protect his roommates, he was moved to a single room in a nearby hotel. A substitute rower took his position in the boat.

Except for common meals, rower B had no direct contact with his teammates. Within five days, his physiological state of health improved, but his mood declined steadily, which was detected during his daily medical treatment. At this point, the staff raised the question whether he should participate in a planned joint day off. The day off activities involved more than just relaxing, as the team members were going to an amusement park and had planned a program that also involved physical effort.

Diagnosis: Just before the day off, the next RESTQ-Sport measurement took place. The RESTQ-Sport profile showed high scores in the *Physical Complaints* scale (figure 3.2). All other stress-related scales showed normal values. At the same time, all recovery-related scores had decreased dramatically. The low scores for *Physical Recovery* were understandable because of the illness of the rower. Due to lack of practice, the decreased scores in the sport-specific areas could also be understood. Obviously, the athlete's lack of or reduced social activity in the preceding three days/nights was responsible for the low scores in all recovery-related areas.

Intervention: After considering the risk for the team and the sick athlete, the head coach and the

medical staff decided that rower B could participate in the day off activities with the team. The risk of total isolation from his teammates and the subsequent impairment of performance ability or other problems upon returning to his position in the boat was rated higher than the risk of impairing rower B's state of health or infecting his teammates. After a few days, rower B could participate in regular practice and regained his position in the boat. Ultimately, the team won the World Championships.

RESTQ-76 Sport Profile:

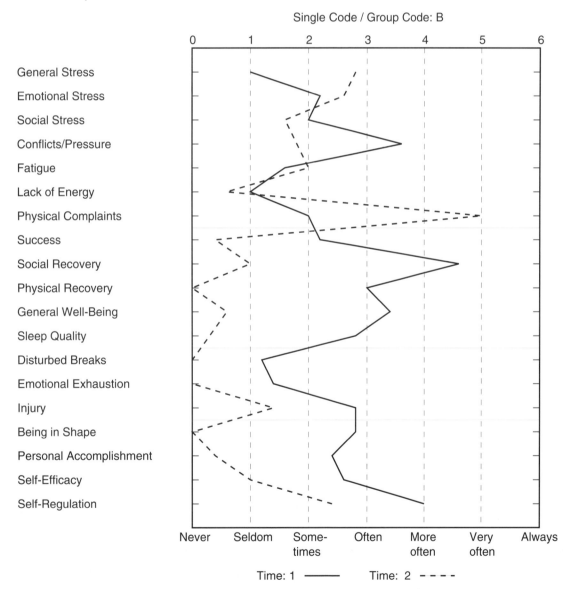

Figure 3.2 RESTQ-Sport profile for the male rower B before (Trial: 1) and after (Trial: 2) illness.

Case 3: Rowers C and D

Description and diagnosis: Two rowers (C and D) were in the same boat, had the same coach, and consequently also had the same training load during training camp. After a day and a half off from practice, which was part of the training schedule, completely different developments were detected for both athletes (figure 3.3, a and b).

For rower C, stress decreased and recovery increased as expected. No large changes occurred for rower D in the stress-related scales, but the scores of the recovery-related fields dropped significantly after the day and a half off.

Intervention: Based on the results, the coach talked to the athletes about possible causes for the decrease in the recovery scales. One consequence was that the training had to be adapted for rower D (i.e., the number of rounds reduced in the weight lifting portion). Knowing that a training reduction for just one person creates an awkward situation, all team members were informed that for the next few days the weight lifting training would be individually adapted, meaning that some athletes would train more than others.

RESTQ-76 Sport Profile:

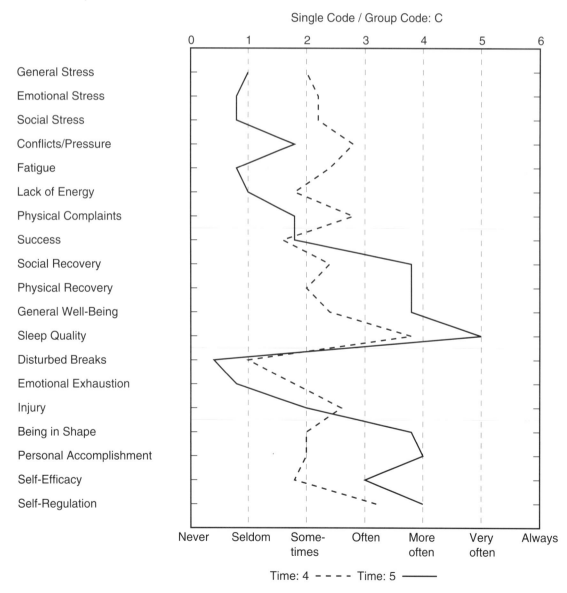

Figure 3.3a Recovery-stress state for rower C at T4 (broken line) and T5 (solid line).

RESTQ-76 Sport Profile:

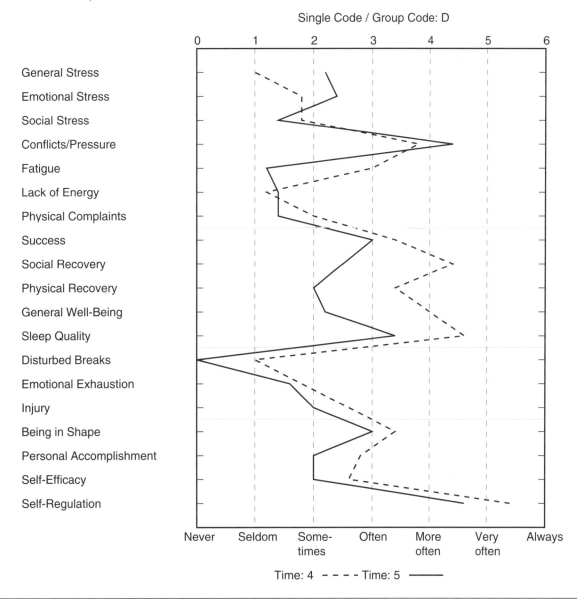

Figure 3.3b   Recovery-stress state for rower D at T4 (broken line) and T5 (solid line).

Case 4: Disturbed Sleep

Description, diagnosis, and intervention: For organizational reasons, some rowers had to move to a nearby hotel during training camp. A subsequent dramatic decrease in the *Sleep Quality* scores of all rowers led the coach to talk to his athletes about the situation and possible sleep-disturbing factors.

The coach learned that the hotel room had a TV, which the athletes were using for relaxation after practice. However, the use of the TV turned out to be the cause for the *Sleep Quality* deficit because the athletes continued to watch it after bedtime and during the recovery periods after lunch. Consequently, the TV was taken out of the room and the scores in *Sleep Quality* increased.

Case 5: Backup for Coaches

Description, diagnosis, and intervention: Because of an injury of the female four-coxed stroke one day before the preliminary heat in the 1997 World Championships, another rower had to take the critical stroke position. The coach based his decision about who would take the important stroke position on the available information from practice as well as performance data; however, he was not totally convinced that he had made the right choice. Therefore, he approached the sport psychological consultant with the following question: "Can I do any harm by putting rower E on the stroke position?" Because all four athletes had previously completed the RESTQ-Sport four times, their profiles could be compared over time. In this case, all information supported the coach's choice, especially that from the sport-specific scales (e.g., *Self-Efficacy, Self-Regulation*). With the replacement rower, the boat won the World Championships.

Case 6: Different Perspectives of Athletes and the Coach

Description, diagnosis, and intervention: This case has to do with events during the 1997 Junior World Championships in Hazewinkel, Belgium. The athletes had completed the RESTQ-Sport five times during the camp and before and after the preliminary heat. The female coxed eight of the German Junior National Rowing Team won their preliminary heat by an outstanding 8 sec, immediately qualifying for the finals.

Before the opening of the World Championships and the first race in an actual competition, some athletes got food poisoning and had to be replaced. Although the athletes and coaches were concerned about the practice program, the positive outcome in the preliminary race relieved some of the pressure by showing that the athletes were well prepared.

The victory was not obvious from the individual recovery-stress state profiles of the coxed eight, however. For key positions such as the stroke, scores for *Self-Efficacy* and *Self-Regulation* were relatively low. The coach was surprised, as all the athletes seemed self-confident and relaxed; having experience with the RESTQ-Sport, he decided to look into the matter. He learned from the stroke that she felt additional pressure and anxiety because expectations for the final race were so high. Whereas most other team members seemed to feel less pressure after the win, she felt added pressure. The coach held an informal meeting to review the victory and addressed the fact that it affected individual rowers differently. The stroke tearfully communicated her feelings, her astonished teammates expressed their concern and support, and another rower divulged her insecurity. The meeting seemed to be another important step in a continuing team-building process. In the finals, the boat performed at the preliminary-heat level and won the World Championships.

Summary

- It must always be kept in mind that the RESTQ-Sport profile reflects just *one short period in a person's life*, which may change drastically within a few days.

- The RESTQ-Sport makes it possible to observe individuals and/or groups during training camp and over the course of a season.

- The RESTQ-Sport identifies athletes whose recovery-stress state does not correspond with changes in the training schedule during training camp.

- Coaches' and athletes' perceptions often differ.

PART II
Theory, Construction, and Validity

CHAPTER 4

Theory

Throughout this chapter the main concepts and the theoretical background for the development of the Recovery-Stress Questionnaire for Athletes are introduced. The definitions of stress and recovery and their interaction will clearly show that stress and recovery need to be assessed by a multilevel approach.

Stress

From a system-oriented viewpoint, stress is a destabilization or deviation from the norm in a biological/psychological system (psychophysical balance). The amount a particular system deviates from its optimal value (desired value) is influenced by specific standards and leads to a desired/actual value discrepancy (e.g., Boucsein, 1991). Deviations from the psychophysical balance are characteristic of demands that are too high and demands that are too low. As a result, fatigue, sleepiness, psychological stress, monotony, or psychological saturation can occur (Hacker & Richter, 1984).

Applied psychology, especially in the seventies, separated the concepts of stress and strain. Stress is considered to be *objective sizes and factors, affecting people from the outside*. Strain is understood to be the result of these stressors on the side of the person; that is, their *effect in people and on people* (Fletcher, 1988; Rohmert & Rutenfranz, 1975). Because of the limited use of the word *strain* in many areas of stress research, throughout this manual the term *stress* will be used to address the person side of the transaction ("strain") and the term *stressor* will be used for the situational aspects. From a psychological viewpoint, the mediating subjective appraisal processes of a person play a predominant role (e.g., Jerusalem, 1990; Lazarus, 1991; Lazarus & Launier, 1978). Depending on the subjective perception of objective facts, the same stressor can cause different stresses. The individual is not passively exposed to the stressors but can influence them in their quality and quantity, depending on the goal of action, and can even induce or avoid them.

Stress can have positive and negative effects, depending on the state of the person and the recovery processes. Stress, coping, and recovery determine the state of the person, which in turn determines the reactions to subsequent stressors (Kallus, 1992). Thus, the recovery-stress state plays a key role in the understanding of stress effects. The recovery-stress state allows taking into account the resources of the person, as resources determine the person's ability to cope with stressors and thus even determine the appraisal of stressors.

According to Schönpflug (1983, 1987) and others, the reactions to stress depend on permanent and consumptive resources, which can offer a person some resistance to stress. Consumptive resources are dependent on regeneration and recovery, whereas permanent resources are dependent on the person's skills and abilities. Consumptive resources (e.g., effort, tension, will, power, and energy with limited reserves and clear proportional reduction) activate, keep up, and support the permanent resources, which include long-term internal performance requirements such as talent, competence, and capacity. Limited capacities, or the inability to refill the consumptive resources, negatively affect the immediate regeneration of the permanent resources. Consequently, the risk of a total exhaustion of resources increases. Therefore, the goal should always be to create, care for, use wisely, repair after use, and replace both consumptive and permanent resources when diminished (Schönpflug, 1987).

Besides the *intensity* of stress, the *duration* and the *distribution in time* determine the necessity of regeneration and recovery. The possible positive consequences of action latitude on stress are also discussed in modern action psychological models (Frese & Zapf, 1994; Schönpflug, 1987) and in publications on the biopsychology of stress (Janke & Wolffgramm, 1995). Stress, as a transactional process in time, can neither be examined nor validly diagnosed without the involvement of adaptation and coping processes, without consideration of the individually observed recovery possibilities, and without involvement of feedback processes of the organism. Although many methods are available for the recording of coping processes (see Rüger, Blomert, & Förster, 1990), there was insufficient assessment of the recovery processes until the construction of the RESTQ.

The interrelation between the baseline condition and stress has been portrayed by Kallus (1992, 1995) as a feedback process. Stress reactions influence the baseline condition, which on its part influences the reactions to stress. The complete model shows that the baseline condition for further stress reactions is influenced by stress, recovery activities, and the method of coping with antecedent stressors. The interrelation between stress and recovery has also been emphasized by Wieland-Eckelmann and Baggen (1994), who introduced the work-recovery cycle. The work-recovery cycle is determined by the (task-related) request/capacity relation, the expense/return relation, the (recovery-related) expense/return relation, and the relation between the need for recovery and the possibility of recovery. "The crucial assumption for successful recovery processes is the relation between the individual ability to recover and the stress consequences resulting from work stress" (Wieland-Eckelmann & Baggen, 1994, p. 105).

Recovery

Many definitions describe recovery as a compensation of deficit conditions of the organism that are activity determined. Often the principle of homeostasis has been taken as an explanatory concept in which recovery supposedly leads to restoration of the baseline condition. For example, Allmer and Niehues (1989) labeled recovery with reference to Renzland and Eberspächer (1988) as a process "through which the psychological consequences of stress from preceding activities are balanced and the individual condition to act is restored" (p. 18). Kallus (1995) and Kallus and Kellmann (2000) describe the complex processes and propose characteristics of a general psychophysiological concept of recovery (table 4.1).

The defining characteristics of recovery show that it is not sufficient to speak only of eliminating fatigue or restarting the system. Only the differentiated and longitudinally oriented observation can reflect the complex individual recovery process. Based on the features of recovery (Kallus, 1995), a more precise definition was developed: *Recovery is an inter- and intraindividual multilevel (e.g., psychological, physiological, social) process in time for the re-establishment of performance abilities. Recovery includes an action-oriented component, and those self-initiated activities (proactive recovery) can be systematically used to optimize situational conditions to build up and to refill personal resources and buffers."*

Table 4.1 Characteristics of Recovery

- Recovery is a process in time.

- Recovery is related to the type of and duration of stress.

- Recovery depends on a reduction of, a change of, or a break from stress.

- Recovery is individually specific and depends on individual appraisal.

- Recovery ends when a psychophyscial state of restored efficiency and homeostatic balance is reached.

- Recovery includes purposeful action (proactive recovery), as well as automated psychological and biological processes restoring the initial state (passive recovery).

- Recovery can be described on various levels (e.g., physiological level, psychological level, social level, sociocultural level, environmental level).

- Recovery processes can be displayed in various organismic subsystems.

- Various subprocesses of recovery can be dissociated.

- Recovery is closely tied to boundary conditions (e.g., sleep, social contact, etc.)

Adapted, by permission, from K.W. Kallus and M. Kellmann, 2000, Burnout in Athletes and Coaches. In *Emotions in Sport*, edited by Y.L. Hanin (Champaign, IL: Human Kinetics), 210.

In sport, the time between two stressors serves for physical and psychological regeneration. Often, the concept of regeneration is unclear and is equated with recreation, restoration, or recovery; however, psychophysical regeneration is an "intentional, planned, and controlled process for creating the best possible subjective conditions to act for coping with upcoming demands following a period of stress" (Renzland & Eberspächer, 1988, p. 15). Therefore, regeneration measures must optimize the psychophysical processes following demands and must put athletes in a position to cope optimally with training and competition demands, in this way increasing their psychological and physiological upper limits.

Recovery processes such as sleep, autonomous heart rate abatement, post-stress changes in blood circulation and metabolism, hormonal changes, and most of all, autonomous recovery activities, are not or are only partially part of the regeneration concept. Kallus (1995) and Kallus, Eberspächer, and Hermann (1992) view recovery as a generic concept that integrates regeneration. Rieder, Riffelt, and Vierneisel (1988) conclude that in addition to physical recovery, there are psychological and cognitive recovery processes, but less is known for certain about their ability to be influenced.

As outlined in table 4.1, recovery is individual-specific and depends on individual appraisals. For example, if you ask 10 people to name their personal number-one recovery strategy, you will get seven or eight different answers. In the sport context, a recovery activity selected by a coach for an entire team will not achieve the desired result in all team members because of individual-specific recovery needs. For example, selecting a sauna as a recovery activity may be very relaxing for some athletes, whereas others may feel uncomfortable in a sauna, perceiving it as a stressor.

Not only must recovery strategies be applied individually, but it is also recommended that each individual have more than one recovery strategy available. Sometimes, the first choice cannot be used or does not work due to external or internal circumstances. For example, a person's number-one recovery strategy of "going for a run" may work perfectly in a familiar environment, but in the first few days after traveling overseas and crossing several time zones, the same recovery activity may stress the organismic systems while the individual is still suffering from jet lag. The result is likely to be more stress instead of recovery. A second, third, or fourth backup recovery strategy should be available and applied, depending on current personal

and situational factors, as it is not always possible to use the number-one recovery strategy (Kellmann, in press).

Recovery processes in competitive sport support the restoration of individual action conditions and well-being following training and competition demands (Allmer, 1996). Optimal use of the available recovery time is imperative for success in sport. Top performances are only to be achieved by athletes who can recover fast during competition (Renzland & Eberspächer, 1988) and optimally carry out the changes between stress, recovery, and upcoming stress. In this connection, Eberspächer (1990, 1995) speaks of the floodgate function of a competition break. This model proposes that the optimal break between two stressful periods (e.g., between two heats) includes three phases: evaluation, transition, and preparation.

The *evaluation phase* enables the athlete to process the results from the first heat and to cope with psychological and physical stress. During this phase, regeneration occurs, and the energy reservoirs are refilled.

The *transitional phase* takes most of the time and serves as recovery. The activities in this phase can take many forms. Eating, drinking, dozing, sleeping, playing cards, meeting friends, or other mostly unplanned activities are typical transitional activities at competitions. There is some doubt, however, as to whether they all bring the desired recovery effect. It is best for each proactive person to develop his own strategy and consciously decide how to make most the effective use of a break. However, deciding on the optimal recovery strategy must take into account individual peculiarities. Whereas some feel recovered after a nap, others are absolutely wiped out. There is no generally valid recipe.

The final phase of a break, the *preparation phase* for the next heat, starts with the physiological warm-up and the mental focusing on the race to restore the performance preparedness of the mind and body.

Interaction Between Stress and Recovery

For working processes and for sport, the kind of stress and the kind of recovery that interact with each other depend on the nature of the activity (Allmer, 1996; Kuipers & Keizer, 1988; Lehmann, Foster, & Keul, 1993; Löhr & Preiser, 1974). Stress can result in overtraining, or in the case of sufficient recovery, in a positive training effect, and in this way stimulate the ability to cope with stress through practice and adjustment processes. More long-term growth in achievement in the sense of a training effect can be achieved by means of a suitable distribution of stress and rest periods over time, with short-term fatigue and overtraining caused by the training followed by recovery (Weineck, 1994). Therefore, a planned, achievement-optimizing control of training integrates systematic recovery times and/or training phases with less intensity. Chronic effects in the psychological and physiological areas can result from ignored recovery (e.g., Budgett, 1998; Foster, 1998; Hoffmann, Epstein, Yarom, Zigel, & Einbinder, 1999; Kellmann, 2000, in press; Kellmann & Günther, 2000; Kellmann et al., 1999; Kuipers, 1998; Lehmann et al., 1993; Lehmann et al., 1997; Lehmann, Foster, Dickhut, & Gastmann, 1998).

To prevent the negative effects of enhanced training intensity, practice has to be well planned and the evaluation of training effects should be included as part of this routine. The basic training affects factors (intensity and volume) that can be described by the speed (or power) and training time (or repetitions, for example). Specific analysis enables the estimation of further parameters such as intensity of stress with heart rate and lactate, the muscular effects with the increase of creatine kinase (CK) or uric acid in the blood, the training volume, and the total training load with urea. With increased effort, the stress reaction can also be assessed on the hormonal level (Lehmann et al., 1993; Steinacker, 1993; Steinacker, Laske, Hetzel, Lormes, Liu, & Strauch, 1993). The measurement of sport medical parameters during training camp are part of the training camp routine (e.g., before the World Championships). However, the verbal interaction between the doctor and the athlete during the sport medical treatment and consultation is often more sensitive so as to detect signs of overtraining/underrecovery as biochemical parameters. An intensive consultation depends on the number of athletes and doctors on the team and, even more important, on the available time budget. Therefore, the use of psychometric instruments such as the RESTQ-Sport can be very economical, and in addition, they have no a priori bias, which often affects the perspective of the consultant.

One goal of research on overtraining and staleness is to determine indicators that sensitively predict such a negative development (Raglin, 1993). In this regard, the Profile of Mood States (McNair, Lorr, & Droppleman, 1971, 1992) and the nonspecific areas of the Recovery-Stress Questionnaire for Athletes seem well qualified. When appropriate feedback is provided to athletes by a trained person—such as a sport psychologist—the scores of the

RESTQ-Sport can enhance self-awareness on how personal activities or events in daily life affect the individual recovery-stress state. In particular, when the questionnaire is completed on a regular basis, the changes over time help to educate athletes that recovery is a key issue and important for their sport career.

Stress States and Recovery Demands

Kellmann (1991, 1997) has proposed a model describing the interrelation between stress states and recovery demands (figure 4.1). The basic assumption is that with increasing stress, increased recovery is necessary. Limited resources (e.g., time) initiate a vicious cycle: under increased stress and the inability to meet increased recovery demands, the athlete experiences more stress. Athletes may be stressed to the point where they fail to find or make time to recover adequately or to consider better ways of coping with the situation.

In this model, the simplest case is a symmetrical increase in stress and recovery demands: the two axes drift apart with elevated stress levels ("scissors" function). With intermediate levels of stress, one can find an area of optimal performance and thus an area of adequate recovery (continuous arrows in figure 4.1). Beyond this point, one cannot meet recovery demands without additional recovery activities. Stress will accumulate, and without intervention, burnout or overtraining symptoms will likely develop (see the discussion of burnout later in this chapter). The state of balanced stress and recovery is related to optimal performance and perhaps to the performance-related psychobiosocial states and their emotional correlations within the Individual Zones of Optimal Functioning (IZOF) model (Hanin, 1997, 2000).

In a state of adequate recovery, the individual can react appropriately and cope successfully with stress without additional recovery activities. Lack of recovery can trigger a process that brings on a state of elevated stress. As increasing stress limits the possibility of recovery, the athlete must be given special opportunities for recovery to reestablish an optimal level of performance (Kallus & Kellmann, 2000; Kellmann, in press). In summary, the model suggests that it is not bad to be high on stress, as long as the individual knows how to recover optimally.

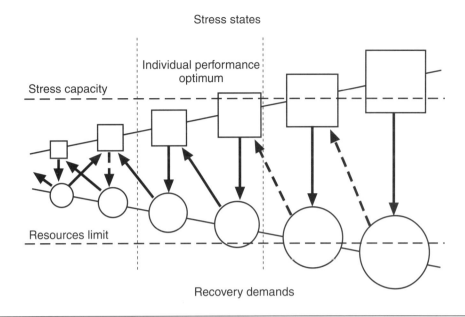

Stress states

Individual performance
optimum

Stress capacity

Resources limit

Recovery demands

Figure 4.1   The "scissors model" of the interrelation between stress states and recovery demands.

Reprinted, by permission, from K.W. Kallus and M. Kellmann, 2000, Burnout in Athletes and Coaches. In *Emotions in Sport*, edited by Y.L. Hanin (Champaign, IL: Human Kinetics), 212.

Sport-Specific Concepts of the Recovery-Stress States

The *break* serves as a phase for psychological (e.g., mental, cognitive, emotional) and physiological regeneration during competition for athletes and for their interaction with coaches and advisors (Anshel, 1997; Hagedorn, 1989; Hahn, 1978). In athletic activity, it is often shown that the athletes are given more information than they can digest during the recovery phase (Herzog, Voigt, & Westphal, 1985). Many coaches are unaware of the meaning of the recovery phase and are not conscious of its correlation with the recovery process. This can result in insufficient or disturbed recovery such as interrupted recovery or an irregular recovery pattern. Insufficient recovery can be the result of too short breaks with an absence of optimal recovery. If the requirements of adequate recovery are present but the athlete is disturbed through other means (i.e., emotional discussion between coach and athlete, noise disturbances), inadequate recovery can nevertheless result. Hahn (1978) considers the continuous mention of players' mistakes during the halftime discussion to be detrimental to the recovery process. Therefore, the coach's behavior plays a central role in the structure of the recovery between stress situations (Kellmann, 1997; Kellmann & Kallus, 1994, 1995). In laboratory experiments, Kallus (see Kallus & Krauth,

1995) indicated that during the regeneration phase, there is a considerable increase in the amount of sensitivity toward disturbances, annoyances, and irritations (Wilhelm & Janssen, 1989). Therefore, slight interruptions in the normal situation during the break may have great effects on an athlete's performance. The recovery phase does not just compensate for exhaustion; it is also a significant preventive measure for stress situations (Hahn, 1987).

For many years, *burnout* has become meaningful in stress research (Schönflug, 1987). Although no common definition for burnout exists (Dale & Weinberg, 1989; Fender, 1989; Pines, 1993; Smith, 1986), it is agreed that burnout is a reaction to chronic stress (Dale & Weinberg, 1989; Maslach & Jackson, 1986; Smith, 1986, 1989). According to Maslach and Jackson (1986), burnout syndrome is apparent through emotional exhaustion, depersonalization, and lack of personal accomplishment. Not only does this have a negative effect on performance, but it also amounts to an increase in the dropout rate of the practiced activities. After research on burnout was carried out in the social professions (Pines, 1993), it was expanded to other professional groups. Next to teachers, athletic trainers were the center of attention in burnout research (see Kallus & Kellmann, 2000). Burnout has definitely been shown to have an effect on athletes. Moreover, with an increase in the degree of burnout, the athlete's performance declines and becomes inconsistent (Cohn, 1990; Smith, 1986). "Burnout in the sport situation will be defined as a reaction to the stresses of athletic competition that can be characterized by feelings of emotional exhaustion, an impersonal attitude toward those the athlete associates with, and decreased athletic performance" (Fender, 1989, p. 64).

Not only is there a connection between the degree of burnout and decreases in performance, but also with increases in dropout. The effect is amplified by overtraining, routine, monotony, boredom, and a lack of diversity (Fender, 1989; Odom & Perrin, 1985; Robinson & Carron, 1982; Smith, 1989). Henschen (1993) believes that burnout is caused by a lack of recovery. Neither psychological nor physiological recovery is possible during an intensive season with a high amount of training during the off-season. According to Henschen (1993), if burnout occurs, the only useful measure is to give the athlete a long recovery phase or a temporary reduction in athletic activities. This can prevent the athlete having to end her athletic career. Therefore, the coach/advisor must be sensitive to the athlete's psychological and/or physical recovery demands and contribute to the maintenance of an optimal recovery-stress state.

Another important aspect of the RESTQ-Sport deals with *self-efficacy*. The concept of self-efficacy is closely related to Bandura (1977). He proved that a person's actions are influenced by the person's expectations of their effectiveness. A person's positive and/or negative expectations of an action determine the duration of the action and the stress intensity (if the action is initiated in a stress situation). The influence of intensity on efficacy expectations depends on how high a person's demands are and how much the person is convinced of an action's effectiveness.

Motivated actions are separated into a cognitive representation of a chain of events (situation-action-outcome-consequences) in which the single elements are closely bound with each other through certain expectations: outcome-consequence-expectation (instrumentality), situation-action-expectation (expected competence), action-outcome-expectation (expected consequence) (Jerusalem, 1990). The expected consequence means that, according to the person's evaluation, a certain action results in a certain outcome. Contrary to the expected competence is a person's conviction of being able to actually use behavior that results in a certain outcome (see Vroom's model of motivation, 1964). The expected competence is also the subjective evaluation of the action's availability and is combined with the expected consequence of the action's execution. Accordingly, the expected consequence is not relevant without the expected competence. Therefore, not only is the knowledge of correct forms of movement necessary to carry out an action successfully, but also the subjective conviction that these motions can be carried out successfully in every situation. Additionally, the instrumentality decides if the outcome is meaningful for higher goals; for example, winning a competition that does not bring a financial reward or points for the ranking list has less instrumentality for a professional athlete.

Self-efficacy has a positive influence on an athlete's performance (Eberspächer & Kellmann, 1997; Feltz, Landers, & Raeder, 1979; George, Feltz, & Chase, 1992; Spink, 1990). The straightforwardness and verification of these results largely correlate with the theoretical fundamentals of this concept. McAuley (1985) and Wittig, Duncan, and Schnurr (1987) reported that the increase in self-efficacy accompanies a reduction in fear, which can also increase the athlete's well-being. Feltz and Riessinger (1990) proved that self-efficacy depends on one's own experience (86%), whereas the information on environmental conditions plays a secondary role. Thus, it is not the information about environmental conditions (i.e., the athletic opponent) that leads to a change in expected competence, but the athlete's expectations, which are based on the athlete's own experience.

Summary

- It is important to create, care for, use wisely, repair after use, and replace *resources* when lost.

- Stress can result in overtraining, or in the case of sufficient recovery, in a positive training effect, and in this way stimulate the ability to cope with stress through practice and adjustment processes.

- A complex interrelation exists between coping, recovery, and adjustment processes.

- Recovery is an inter- and intraindividual multilevel process in time for the reestablishment of performance abilities.

- Recovery includes an action-oriented component, and those self-initiated activities can be systematically used to optimize situational conditions to build up and refill personal resources and buffers.

- Top performances are only achieved by athletes who can recover fast during competition and deal optimally with the changes between stress, recovery, and upcoming stress.

- Insufficient recovery can be the result of too short breaks with an absence of optimal recovery.

- It is not bad to be high on stress, as long as the individual knows how to recover optimally.

CHAPTER 5

Construction of the Recovery-Stress Questionnaire for Athletes

The Recovery-Stress Questionnaire for Athletes follows the construction principle of Kallus (1995), which included, on the one hand, a precise subjective appraisal of events in the assessment and, on the other hand, an accurate focus on the frequency of behavior. This objective was attained by focusing on frequencies of events, activities, and states in the past three days/nights by pretending to *appraise* events using statements such as *I had a good time with friends* instead of *I met some friends*.

Claim to Validity of the Recovery-Stress Questionnaire for Athletes

The approach of using appraised events was continued with the development of the sport-specific RESTQ scales. The construction and validation of the questionnaire were based on the following requirements:

- The RESTQ-Sport scales should provide comparable psychometric values of the general RESTQ and should follow its construction principle.
- The scale should display an internal consistency above α > .7.
- The factorial structure of the RESTQ-Sport should match the general RESTQ. The sport-specific recovery scales should highly load on a recovery factor and the sport-specific stress scales on a stress factor.
- The RESTQ-Sport should provide relatively stable results over a period of a few days (high reliability for test repetition for short time periods). The stability of these results will decrease with time.

- The RESTQ-Sport should be functional in longitudinal designs.
- The questionnaire should sensitively assess the recovery-stress state and reliably monitor changes over different training and competition cycles (training monitoring).
- The RESTQ-Sport should allow for prediction of the intensity of the current training and performance conditions on the basis of the frequency of past stress and recovery situations.
- Relationships are to be expected between the recovery-stress state and intraindividual fluctuations in performance.
- The questionnaire should be usable in different sports and represent differences in the recovery-stress states in various groups of people.
- The questionnaire should clearly represent systematic changes in stress states. This requirement results from the representation of intraindividual deviations of various groups of stressed subjects.

Development of the Recovery-Stress Questionnaire for Athletes

This section describes the development of the Recovery-Stress Questionnaire for Athletes and documents the modifications of the different versions. Tests of reliability and validity in every version ensured the fulfillment of psychometric requirements. Table 5.1 gives an overview of the different RESTQ-Sport versions, scales, and numbers of items

Table 5.1 Scales, Number of Items, Year of Development for the Sport-Specific RESTQ Versions

	RESTQ-Sport scales	1992 86	1995 85	1999 80	1999 76	2000 52
1	General Stress	4	4	4	4	2
2	Emotional Stress	4	4	4	4	2
3	Social Stress	4	4	4	4	2
4	Conflicts/Pressure	4	4	4	4	2
5	Fatigue	4	4	4	4	2
6	Lack of Energy	4	4	4	4	2
7	Physical Complaints	4	4	4	4	2
8	Success	4	4	4	4	2
9	Social Recovery	4	4	4	4	2
10	Physical Recovery	4	4	4	4	2
11	General Well-Being	4	4	4	4	2
12	Sleep Quality	4	4	4	4	2
13	Disturbed Breaks	2	6	4	4	4
14	Emotional Exhaustion	6	4	4	4	4
15	Injury	6	6	4	4	4
16	Being in Shape	6	4	4	4	4
17	Personal Accomplishment	6	5	4	4	4
18	Self-Efficacy	–	6	4	4	4
19	Self-Regulation	12	6	4	4	4
Additional items				4		
Total		86	85	80	76	52

for each scale. An overview of the actual items and scales are provided in appendix table A1.

During an academic year abroad via exchange, the English version of the general Recovery-Stress Questionnaire was used for the first time in a sport-specific context (Kellmann, 1991). A study was conducted with the track and field team of Appalachian State University in North Carolina (U.S.A.) to determine whether the translated version met the psychometric requirements. To assess stress and recovery in sports more specifically, the RESTQ was modified and extended. A second study with different sport teams at Appalachian State University further validated the English sport-specific version.

The First Version: RESTQ-86 Sport

The first version of the RESTQ-Sport is based on the RESTQ-48 plus an additional 38 items in six scales. The new items were lined up randomly and attached to the general RESTQ (see the "Sport-Specific RESTQ Module" section). This supplementary approach results in the modular construction of the RESTQ with different subject-specific forms: RESTQ-Rehabilitation, RESTQ-Work (see Kallus, 1995), and RESTQ-Coach (see Kallus & Kellmann, 1995; Kallus, Kellmann, Eberspächer, & Hermann, 1996).

Development of the sport-specific scales was based on current research in sport psychology and the results of reliability analysis by Kellmann (1991). During the analysis of the various items, it became obvious, for example, that the conceptualization of *Physical Complaints* and *Physical Recovery* seemed too general for athletes. These scales measure physical complaints and relaxation for the general population, but not for athletes where more sport-specific questions are needed; however, for the performance ability of an athlete, physical fitness is a key factor. If the physical conditions are not optimally set up or injuries occur, the quality of performance is limited. Therefore, the *Fitness/Being in Shape* and *Fitness/Injury* scales were constructed with six items each to reflect the physical fitness of an athlete.

As Kallus and Kellmann (2000) pointed out, burnout is an important factor in sports. Based on the Maslach Burnout Inventory (MBI) (Maslach & Jackson, 1986), the most important aspects of the *Burnout/Emotional Exhaustion* and *Burnout/Personal Accomplishment* scales were included in the RESTQ-Sport with six items each. Fender (1989) has stated that the MBI can be used to assess burnout in athletes. Based on the frequency-based format of the MBI, selected items were adapted to the RESTQ-Sport item format.

The 12 items in the *Self-Regulation* scale assess psychological skills (self-talk, attention and activation regulation, imagery, self-efficacy, goal setting, and analysis) described by Eberspächer (1990, 1995). Additionally, the *Breaks* scale measures two items: the conscious use of rest periods and the susceptibility to being disturbed.

RESTQ-85 Sport

The RESTQ-85 Sport consisted of the RESTQ-48 plus the attached 37 items. The *Self-Efficacy* scale was used for the first time (table 5.1). To avoid misunderstanding as to whether the sport-specific items are related to practice or to competition, a general directive was provided in the instructions:

The statements related to performance should refer to performance during competition as well as during practice. To further avoid confusion, some items were marginally modified from the prior version. For example, the statement *I had muscle pain after practice* changed to *I had muscle pain after performance.* Current research on self-efficacy (Bandura, 1977; Eberspächer, Kellmann, & Hermann, 1996; Eberspächer & Kellmann, 1997) recommended a separate assessment, and therefore it was taken out of the *Self-Regulation* scale and became a separate scale. Supplementary items changed the focus of the *Breaks* scale to *Disturbed Breaks.* All sport-specific items were randomized following the procedure described later in the "Sport-Specific RESTQ Module" section.

RESTQ-76 Sport/RESTQ-80 Sport

Based on the reliability procedure for the item analysis and additional psychometric data, the sport-specific scales were shortened to four items for each scale. This final order of the sport-specific scales was randomized following the procedure described in the "Sport-Specific RESTQ Module" section. The RESTQ-76 Sport consists of 19 scales with four items for each scale. Depending on specific research questions, two supplementary items were added for *Self-Efficacy* and *Disturbed Breaks*, making a version with 80 items available for specific studies.

The Final Version: RESTQ-76 Sport/RESTQ-52 Sport

The RESTQ-76 Sport (48 nonspecific and 28 sport-specific items) and the RESTQ-52 Sport (24 nonspecific and 28 sport-specific items) are the product of continuous development over many years. The use of the RESTQ-76 Sport is recommended when only a few measurements can be examined. The RESTQ-52 Sport is recommended in longitudinal designs or when the information in the general scales of the RESTQ-Sport is not the focus of interest. Ideally, a combination of both versions takes place in longitudinal studies (e.g., RESTQ-76 Sport, RESTQ-52 Sport, RESTQ-76 Sport), because all sport-specific items and 24 nonspecific items are included in both versions.

Test Construction

The RESTQ-Sport and the RESTQ are based on the assumption that the current state of stress can be revealed through a person's retrospective data regarding the frequency with which stressful situations and the corresponding reactions, recovery activities, and recovery situations arise in the past three days/nights. In the first version, Kallus (1995) chose a nonspecific time period for the heading of the questionnaire (*in the past few days*). In this way, long-term stress with very definite effects and the related subjective units of time could also be included. However, large variances in the time of reference suggested that the time period should be more clearly defined.

Self-evaluations regarding reactions in various areas (state of health and physical reactions, as well as areas of behavior and performance) are taken into consideration as sources of information. The effects of generalized self-portrayal, influences in the sense of social acceptance and personality traits that are stable over time, and attitudes are expected to be reduced by the preference of behaviorally oriented, frequency-scaled items. In addition to behaviorally oriented items, the area of subjective well-being covers a comparatively broad spectrum; this corresponds with the meaning of subjective appraisal for the occurrence of stress in a multitude of models (Janke, 1976; Kallus, 1992; Laux, 1983; Lazarus & Launier, 1978).

Outline of Item Classification, Item Selection, and Scale Development

The basic RESTQ module and the RESTQ-Sport were constructed according to the principles of classic test theory (Lienert, 1969; Lienert & Raatz, 1994). Due to the objective *prediction of stress reaction* in the item selection, both item variance and corrected item total correlations were included, as well as indices of item validity with regard to stress indicators (current psychological state, blood pressure, and heart rate under experimentally induced stress). As a result, an instrument was created that attempts to achieve high internal consistency; however, that has not been the only criterion for judging the quality of the scales (Gulliksen technique; Lienert, 1969).

Basic RESTQ Module

In accordance with the classification of stressors by Janke (1976), stress and recovery were included in the RESTQ for the following areas: (a) nonspecific events, (b) emotional reactions, (c) social activities, (d) work performance, and (e) physical symptoms. On the basis of this theoretical classification, an item

pool was compiled that should reflect the stress and recovery for each of these areas. Since physiological changes are only accessible by self-evaluation to a limited extent, and are only reflected by physiological malfunction with greater intensity of stress, questions about this area are comparatively underrepresented (Kallus, 1995). Items were selected from an extensive list of observations on various stress and recovery activities, according to the criterion of sufficient frequency of occurrence. The overrepresentation of the area of stress is also due to the initial set of items. This greater emphasis on the area of stress is intended to represent the area of stress reliably, differentially, and selectively. The area of recovery was rated as a significant moderating variable when the questionnaire was first constructed.

Sport-Specific RESTQ Module

The development of the athlete-oriented scales is a continuation of the basic RESTQ. The first draft was developed by using the ad hoc form of a questionnaire. Taking into consideration the apparent validity and scale development, experts used a rational item analysis and chose from a collection of items that demonstrated aspects of stress and recovery (Sprung & Sprung, 1987; also see Krauth, 1995).

The first draft contains a different number of items from the underlying model, depending on homogeneity or heterogeneity. The 38 items of the six scales were numbered by chance (see Kellmann, 1997). The scales were randomly ordered and were further reordered after each round. Finally, for every sequence, an item was randomly pulled to be inserted into the next questionnaire number. The process was repeated until all items were sorted. In The RESTQ-86 Sport, the *Self-Regulation* scale contains two areas with six different cognitive skills each, or a total of 12 items. This was the second independent scale to be chosen randomly. This process imparted a random order to the items with their sequence of numbers. In addition, it ensured that subsequent items did not frequently come from the same scale. This process minimized the risk of damaging an item's local stochastic independence (Krauth, 1995).

The finalized sport-specific scale sequence of the RESTQ-76 Sport and RESTQ-52 Sport is based on intercorrelation and graphic presentation of profiles. To maintain the chronology of the basic RESTQ, the first step was the area of sport-specific stress and was followed by the area of recovery.

Summary

- The RESTQ-Sport includes a precise subjective appraisal of events in the assessment and an accurate focus on the frequency of behavior.

- Self-evaluations regarding reactions from areas such as state of health and physical reactions, as well as areas of behavior and performance, are taken into consideration as sources of information.

- The RESTQ-Sport was constructed according to the principles of classical test theory.

- The RESTQ-76 Sport and the RESTQ-52 Sport are the product of a continuous development over many years.

- The use of the RESTQ-76 Sport is recommended when only a few measurements can be examined. The RESTQ-52 Sport is recommended in longitudinal designs or when the information of the general scales of the RESTQ-Sport is not the focus of interest. Ideally, a combination of both versions takes place in longitudinal studies.

CHAPTER 6

Test Statistics

The construction of the RESTQ-Sport, which began in the United States, was an iterative process that took more than 10 years and involved numerous athletic research samples. The development of the English and German versions of the RESTQ-Sport was dependent on our access to athletic samples and work capacity; however, we managed to carry out an almost parallel development for both languages.

Research Samples

Based on the research samples shown in table 6.1, test statistics as well as reliability and validity were calculated. Three different groups of samples can be found in the table. The American samples (A1-A4) are described in the first part, followed by the Canadian samples (C1-C2). Since some remarkable validity results emerged that were not assessed by the English version, other samples from the German Junior National Rowing Teams (R1-R4) and one additional German sample (G1) have also been included into the analysis. Table 6.1 is an overview of the research samples and the variations of the RESTQ-Sport employed.

Reliability

The general part of the RESTQ-Sport is based on the RESTQ-48, which consists of 24 items that parallel both versions of the RESTQ-24 (A and B). Kallus (1995) introduced this short version in the RESTQ manual using 48 items and pointed out that it is sufficiently reliable and valid for research purposes.

Homogeneity

For the majority of the RESTQ-Sport scales, an overview of the reliability coefficients (table 6.2) shows good to satisfactory estimations of the accuracy of measurement based on the homogeneity of the scales. In contrast to other scales, *Emotional Stress, Lack of Energy, Physical Complaints, Physical Recovery,* and *Disturbed Breaks* show fluctuations in the internal consistencies over the displayed samples.

Consistent with earlier findings, the internal consistencies of the *Conflicts/Pressure, Success* and *Burnout/ Personal Accomplishment* scales turned out to be slightly below Cronbach $\alpha = .7$ (table 6.2), and depending on the sample, the interpretation for those scales is limited. As Kallus (1995) pointed out, the meaning of the general formulated dimension, such as *I finished important tasks,* is different for athletes compared to non-athletes. Also, the item *I had some good ideas* from the *Success* scale is mostly irrelevant for athletes during daily practice because they have to follow the instructions of the coach. *Good ideas* are not important in daily practice. A similar situation exists for *Conflicts/Pressure* (i.e., *I felt I had to perform well in front of others; I felt under pressure*), where the relevance differs depending on the time of assessment. The statements have a different meaning when the RESTQ-Sport is completed after the selection trials for the national team compared to midway during training camp. The importance of *Conflicts/Pressure* increases when the World Championships approach, which is usually reflected by a clear increase of Cronbach α. It must be noted that *Burnout/Personal Accomplishment* includes two items referring to teammates. Since most of the subjects in the American and Canadian samples came from individual sports, the term *teammate* may be used differently. In German samples, the Cronbach α is much higher if athletes from team sports are involved. In general, with large samples, either an analysis of the internal consistency is recommended before interpretation or the *Conflicts/Pressure, Success,* and *Burnout/Personal Accomplishment* scales should be interpreted cautiously.

The satisfactory but not outstanding internal consistencies for *Physical Complaints* indicate that this scale may not be sufficiently sensitive for athletes. This interpretation is supported by the high Cronbach α for the physically oriented sport-specific fitness scales, *Being in Shape* and *Injury.* Obviously, these items assess the athletes'

Table 6.1 Research Samples (American [A], Canadian [C], and German [R,G] Used to Test Validity and Reliability

	A1	A2	A3	A4	C1	C2
Author/ year	Kellmann, 1990	Kellmann, 1992	Martin, Wrisberg, 1995	Kellmann, Johnson, Wrisberg, 1995	Kellmann et al., 1999	Kellmann et al., 1999
Sample size	$n = 33$	$n = 91$	$n = 81$	$n = 23$	$n = 88$	$n = 128$
Gender distribution	Male = 13 Female = 20	Male = 43 Female = 48	Male = 28 Female = 53	Male = 0 Female = 23	Male = 35 Female = 51 ni = 2	Male = 65 Female = 63
Sport	Track and field	Various sports	Golf/swimming	Swimming	Various sports	Various sports
Age	$M = 20.00$ $SD = 1.00$ $R = 18 - 23$	$M = 19.65$ $SD = 1.45$ $R = 13 - 23$	$M = $ ni $SD = $ ni $R = 18 - 22$	$M = 19.43$ $SD = 1.25$ $R = 18 - 23$	$M = 23.68$ $SD = 3.78$ $R = 18 - 38$	$M = 21.82$ $SD = 3.55$ $R = 16 - 33$
RESTQ version	RESTQ	RESTQ-86 Sport	RESTQ-85 Sport	RESTQ-85 Sport	RESTQ-80 Sport	RESTQ-76 Sport
Time frame	3 days/nights	3 days/nights	3 days/nights	3 days/nights	3 days/nights	3 days/nights
Measurements	5	1	1	3	1	1
Instruments	RESTQ, STAI	RESTQ-Sport, STAI, SCI	RESTQ-Sport	RESTQ-Sport, POMS	RESTQ-Sport, POMS, SCI	RESTQ-Sport
Special features	Performance data		Performance data	Performance data		

	R1	R2	R3	R4	G1
Author/ year	Kellmann et al., 1995	Kellmann et al., 1996	Kellmann et al., 1997	Kellmann et al., 1998	Kellmann, Beckmann, 1998
Sample size	n = 42	n = 45	n = 62	n = 58	n = 93
Gender distribution	Male = 28 Female = 14	Male = 22 Female = 23	Male = 37 Female = 25	Male = 33 Female = 25	Male = 42 Female = 36 ni = 19
Sport	JNT-Rowing	JNT-Rowing	JNT-Rowing	JNT-Rowing	Various sports
Age	M = 17.45 SD = 0.71 R = 16 - 18	M = 17.24 SD = 0.74 R = 15 - 18	M = 17.15 SD = 0.85 R = 15 - 18	M = 17.1 SD = 0.72 R = 16 - 18	M = 23.69 SD = 5.68 R = 14 - 44
RESTQ version	RESTQ-80 Sport	RESTQ-80 Sport	RESTQ-80 Sport	RESTQ-76 Sport	RESTQ-76 Sport
Time frame	3 days/nights	3 days/nights	3 days/nights	3 days/nights	3 days/nights
Measurements	5	5	5	9	1
Instruments	RESTQ-Sport, MPSL	RESTQ-Sport	RESTQ-Sport	RESTQ-Sport, VCQ, RESTQ-24, POMS	RESTQ-Sport, VCQ, POMS
Special features	Sport medical data, performance data	Sport medical data, performance data	Sport medical data, performance data	Sport medical data, performance data	

n = sample size
R = range
M = mean
SD = standard deviation
ni = no information

POMS = Profile of Mood States
VCQ = Volitional Component Questionnaire
MPSL = Multidimensional Physical Symptom List
JNT = Junior National Team
SCI = German Stress Coping Inventory
STAI = State-Trait Anxiety Inventory
RESTQ-Sport = Recovery-Stress Questionnaire for Athletes
American (A), Canadian (C), and German samples (R, G)

Table 6.2 Estimation of Reliability (Cronbach α) for the RESTQ-Sport for American (A2, A3), Canadian (C1, C2), and German (R1-3) Samples

						Cronbach α	
Samples						R1-3	R1-3
		A2	A3	C1	C2	1. time	2. time
RESTQ-Sport scales		$n = 87$	$n = 81$	$n = 88$	$n = 128$	$n = 149$	$n = 149$
1	General Stress	.87	.82	.85	.91	.75	.76
2	Emotional Stress	.74	.63	.83	.84	.66	.71
3	Social Stress	.83	.85	.83	.90	.80	.85
4	Conflicts/Pressure	.58	.66	.76	.80	.55	.68
5	Fatigue	.78	.86	.81	.82	.71	.78
6	Lack of Energy	.82	.63	.66	.83	.58	.72
7	Physical Complaints	.77	.66	.71	.78	.71	.71
8	Success	.71	.54	.66	.78	.53	.67
9	Social Recovery	.78	.77	.82	.86	.76	.80
10	Physical Recovery	.71	.61	.77	.83	.77	.85
11	General Well-Being	.85	.88	.92	.93	.84	.84
12	Sleep Quality	.71	.83	.88	.86	.81	.83
13	Disturbed Breaks	—	<.50	.61	.83	.65	.79
14	Emotional Exhaustion	.78	.81	.76	.86	.65	.71
15	Injury	.72	.82	.83	.82	.73	.78
16	Being in Shape	.75	.85	.86	.87	.80	.88
17	Personal Accomplishment	.62	.67	.69	.72	.67	.80
18	Self-Efficacy	—	.92	.88	.88	.84	.89
19	Self-Regulation	.85	.78	.82	.83	.81	.83

situations more sensitively and are more relevant to daily practice than the general formulations for non-athletes.

Table 6.2 contains the changes in homogeneity of the RESTQ-Sport for the pooled samples (R1-3) of the German Junior National Rowing Team from 1995 to 1997. For the first measurement, the Cronbach α are lower compared to the second measurement. As a rule, internal consistency increases with the subjects' familiarity with the instrument. Consequently, an introductory measurement is recommended for the applied use, as well as for research questions, so that athletes get to know the RESTQ-Sport. This finding applies not only to the RESTQ-Sport but to questionnaires in general ("Socrates-effect"; Jagodzinski, Kühnel, & Schmidt, 1987). This fundamental problem of changes in the internal consistencies of questionnaire studies receives little attention and is rarely taken into account in research designs. In repeated measurement studies, changes can be assumed to occur in the responses of the subjects. For example, with performance tests, it is standard procedure to have an introductory test because of the training effect in repeated measurements (Debus & Janke, 1978).

Test-Retest Reliability

Kallus (1995) has shown that the test-retest reliability of all general stress and recovery scales is quite high after 24 hours for an instrument that records variable states. This is also true for scales that only showed a satisfactory internal consistency, as in the case of *Physical*

Complaints and *Physical Recovery*. The consistently high short-term stability, however, clearly shows the reliability of the procedure. The test-retest reliability always lies clearly above $r = .79$, which implies that intraindividual differences in the recovery-stress states can be well reproduced. Moreover, the high test-retest reliability shows that the results of the RESTQ are stable concerning short-term functionary fluctuations and minor short-term changes in recovery-stress state.

Table 6.3 displays the test-retest reliability of the RESTQ-Sport after 3, 4, 9, 17, and 37 days for the

Table 6.3 Test-Retest Reliability of the RESTQ-Sport Referring to the Past Three Days/ Nights in Various Time Spans for the German Sample R4 ($n = 58$)

| RESTQ-Sport scales | Time between testing intervals | | | | |
	3 days	4 days	9 days	17 days	37 days
1 General Stress	.71	.68	.57	.42	.13
2 Emotional Stress	.72	.63	.55	.19	.12
3 Social Stress	.77	.55	.62	.29	.43
4 Conflicts/Pressure	.73	.78	.72	.46	.30
5 Fatigue	.81	.71	.56	.24	.19
6 Lack of Energy	.68	.63	.52	.36	.18
7 Physical Complaints	.76	.67	.51	.23	.10
8 Success	.70	.81	.62	.26	.19
9 Social Recovery	.74	.74	.60	.48	.35
10 Physical Recovery	.79	.81	.52	.69	.51
11 General Well-Being	.61	.76	.61	.41	.44
12 Sleep Quality	.70	.63	.56	.39	.43
13 Disturbed Breaks	.64	.64	.44	.39	.12
14 Emotional Exhaustion	.72	.70	.51	.53	.31
15 Injury	.59	.77	.65	.50	.16
16 Being in Shape	.71	.77	.63	.58	.45
17 Personal Accomplishment	.81	.62	.58	.49	.42
18 Self-Efficacy	.82	.84	.71	.70	.62
19 Self-Regulation	.77	.74	.76	.51	.42

German sample R4. Test-retest reliabilities were calculated for six measurements, and those that best demonstrate the changes over time are listed in table 6.3.

These results replicate the findings of Kellmann (1991), who stated that the test-retest reliability declines over longer time periods corresponding with the measurement intent of the RESTQ-Sport. Only the *Self-Efficacy* scale remains relatively stable over time.

Construct Validity

Construct validity has been studied with respect to the intercorrelations of scales, the factorial structure, and the stability of the intercorrelations across different samples. Relationships to mood states, volitional components, and other criteria are covered later in the section on criterion validity.

Scale Intercorrelations

The height of the scale intercorrelations proved to be only partially stable across different samples; however, the fundamental correlation pattern is almost unchanged across all samples with respect to stress and recovery areas. Both the stress and the recovery scales correlate positively with the scales of the related areas, but they have a negative relationship with the scales of the opposite areas. This pattern is mainly stable in the comparison between different samples (table 6.4, a-b), genders (table 6.5), and levels of familiarity with the instrument (table 6.6); however, the correlations for males and females of sample C2 deviate slightly from the pattern described above.

The possible moderating variables, gender and familiarity, do not seem to influence the relationship between the scales. The height of the correlations does not necessarily increase with experience in completing the questionnaire (see table 6.6, first vs. second measurement). In addition, no pattern-oriented differences of the correlations can be detected for females or for males.

Factorial Structure of the Scales

Since factor analysis has established itself as a classic instrument for describing the intercorrelational structure, the results will be displayed briefly. With regard to the modular construction of the RESTQ-Sport, the factor analyses were performed separately for the general and the sport-specific parts. Responses to the items of samples A3, C1, and C3 were factor analyzed via Principal Component Analysis followed by a varimax rotation. After the stop criterion (eigenvalue <1; Kaiser), two factors could be extracted for the general as well as for the sport-specific parts of the RESTQ-Sport (table 6.7, a-c).

The results confirm the two-factor solution published by Kallus (1995). All factor analyses suggest one stress-related and one recovery-related factor (table 6.7, a-c). Whereas sample C2 displays a clear two-factor solution, for samples A3 and C1, additional loadings appear. In particular, the negative factor loadings of *Sleep Quality* increases on the stress-related factor. High negative loading in C1 also holds for some recovery scales in the stress-related factor. The general stress-related factor explains approximately 50% of the variance. The recovery-related factor ranges between 13% and 27%. Worth mentioning is the sample-dependent-explained variance; for example, in sample A3, the recovery-related factor explains 13% of the variance; in sample C2, it is 27%.

In general, it can be concluded that the two-factor solution clearly separates the general scales of the RESTQ-Sport into one stress-related and one recovery-related factor.

For the sport-specific scales in all samples, two-factor solutions revealed which can be clearly separated into one stress- and one recovery-related factor (table 6.8, a-c). The sport-specific stress factor (*Disturbed Breaks, Emotional Exhaustion, Injury*) explains about 25% of the variance; the recovery factor (*Being in Shape, Personal Accomplishment, Self-Efficacy, Self-Regulation*) explains approximately 45%. In summary, the sport-specific recovery-related factor explains a higher amount of variance. However, for the interpretation of the %-values for the general and sport-specific scales, it is important to note that stress and recovery factors are based on different numbers of scales.

Criterion Validity of the RESTQ-Sport

The recovery-stress state could be validated against a broad range of criteria, which cover psychological measures such as mood state, classical criteria such as performance, and biological state indicators.

Correlations With Actual Condition/State

The expected relationships between the actual state and the RESTQ-Sport have been empirically verified, which supports the validity of the RESTQ-Sport. Correspondingly, Kallus (1995) published correlations between the general RESTQ and various mood dimensions of the adjective checklist (Eigenschaftwörterliste (EWL); Janke & Debus, 1978). Although the RESTQ and the EWL differ in item format and reference period, the high validity coefficients referring to the actual state can be partly explained by state-oriented questions in the RESTQ.

For the RESTQ-Sport, the link to the actual physical state has been covered by the correlation with the Multidimensional Physical Symptom List (MPSL) (Erdmann & Janke, 1981), the Profile of Mood States (POMS) (McNair, Lorr, & Droppleman, 1971, 1992), and the State-Trait-Anxiety Inventory (STAI) (Spielberger, Gorsuch, & Lushene, 1970). The MPSL measures various physiological processes and complaints. Based on these items, the subjects should rate how they currently feel. The MPSL *General Physical Oversensitivity* scale highly correlates with the physically oriented RESTQ-Sport scales (table 6.9). Here the positive correlations with *Physical Complaints* and *Fitness/Injury* and the negative relationships with *Physical Recovery* and *Fitness/Being in Shape* are obvious. The highest correlations with *Stressed Respiration* are shown for *General Stress, Emotional Stress, Lack of Energy, Physical Complaints,* and the sport-specific stress-related scales, *Disturbed Breaks, Emotional Exhaustion,* and *Injury.*

The original English version of the POMS (McNair et al., 1971, 1992) is a 65-item Likert-format questionnaire with scales ranging from 1 (not at all) to 4 (extremely). The POMS provides a measure of general mood disturbances and six mood states *(Tension, Depression, Anger, Vigor, Fatigue, Confusion).* To match the results of the RESTQ-Sport and the POMS, the time frame in the heading of the POMS was changed to *in the past (3) days/nights* based on the suggestion by McNair et al. (1992).

Although the RESTQ-Sport and the POMS apply different types of scales - frequency vs. intensity (Diener & Emmons, 1984) - analysis revealed close and theoretically expected correlation patterns that matched the results of various German and American samples presented by Kellmann (1999), Kellmann et al. (2001), Kellmann and Günther (2000), as well as Kellmann and Kallus (2000). *Tension, Depression, Anger, Fatigue,* and *Confusion* negatively correlate with recovery-related scales, whereas for *Vigor,* a positive relationship occurs (sample C1, table 6.10). The stress-related RESTQ-Sport scales show a positive interrelation with *Tension, Depression, Anger, Fatigue,* and *Confusion* but a negative interrelation with *Vigor.*

Interestingly, for *Vigor,* the correlation with the recovery-related scales is higher compared to the stress-related scales.

A clear pattern was also found for the recovery and stress-related scales and anxiety measured by the State-Trait Anxiety Inventory (STAI) (Spielberger et al., 1970). A positive correlation was found between stress and anxiety and a negative correlation between anxiety and recovery (table 6.11). A similar correlation has been found in state and trait anxiety in different samples.

Relationships to Motivational Components

The correlation between the current state of stress and different motivational components is shown in table 6.12. The Volitional Component Questionnaire (VCQ) (Kuhl & Fuhrmann, 1998) measures individual differences in volitional or self-regulatory abilities. Generally, this questionnaire can measure how susceptible individuals are, for example, to becoming alienated from their own preferences. From the original 32 VCQ scales, 12 were chosen as relevant for the current results pertaining to athletics. At first sight, the correlations follow the POMS-RESTQ pattern, which has already been described. Negative correlations exist with the general and sport-specific areas of stress and the positive components of volitional control. These positive components positively correlate with the recovery areas. The negative components of volitional control show the opposite.

On closer look, it becomes apparent that the relationships between the general and sport-specific areas of recovery and the positive components of volitional control are considerably higher than in the area of stress. The correlations between the *Positive Self-Motivation, Emotion Control, Self-Relaxation, Initiative,* and *Volitional Self-Efficacy* scales and the RESTQ-Sport *Physical Recovery, Being in Shape, Self-Efficacy,* and *Self-Regulation* scales are almost all above $r > .4$. The relation with the *General Stress, Sleep Quality,* and *Personal Accomplishment* areas are somewhat lower and not quite as consistent. The negative components of volitional control show another pattern. The *Susceptibility to Intrusions, Alienation, Rumination,* and *Passive Avoidance* scales correlate beyond $r > .4$ with the RESTQ-Sport *General Stress* scale. *Susceptibility to Intrusions* also correlates beyond $r > .4$ with the RESTQ-Sport *Emotional* and *Social Stress, Conflicts/Pressure,* and *Lack of Energy* scales.

Recovery-Stress State Patterns

Frequency of stress and recovery have repeatedly been proven to independent dimensions (Kallus, 1995). Two

Table 6.4a Intercorrelation of the RESTQ-86 Sport Scales for the American Samples A2 (*n* = 87) and A3 (*n* = 77)

Upper data matrix: A3

RESTQ Scales	1	2	3	4	5	6	7	8	9	10	11	12	13	14	15	16	17	18	19
1 General Stress		.68	.66	.55	.58	.61	.67	−.11	−.49	−.49	−.64	−.54	.30	.40	.33	−.40	−.24	−.38	−.25
2 Emotional Stress	.78		.70	.60	.42	.51	.55	−.04	−.36	−.33	−.57	−.52	.23	.43	.38	−.18	−.05	−.12	−.05
3 Social Stress	.70	.81		.40	.46	.46	.54	−.12	−.28	−.31	−.52	−.43	.24	.45	.43	−.24	−.24	−.21	−.04
4 Conflicts/Pressure	.58	.57	.48		.41	.51	.40	.20	−.22	−.25	−.34	−.36	.24	.36	.29	−.06	.07	−.07	.14
5 Fatigue	.46	.49	.45	.59		.55	.67	−.13	−.27	−.39	−.36	−.46	.33	.25	.37	−.43	−.16	−.31	−.29
6 Lack of Energy	.64	.63	.50	.60	.44		.54	−.21	−.28	−.44	−.43	−.47	.34	.23	.28	−.32	−.13	−.32	−.26
7 Physical Complaints	.64	.67	.58	.49	.53	.49		−.09	.36	−.52	−.56	−.51	.43	.45	.45	−.52	−.28	−.49	−.29
8 Success	−.37	−.19	−.27	.02	−.05	−.21	−.19		.27	.43	.33	.24	−.22	−.07	.05	.28	.32	.46	.41
9 Social Recovery	−.41	−.41	−.50	−.16	−.16	−.27	−.31	.50		.49	.72	.31	−.11	−.20	−.12	.42	.24	.34	.21
10 Physical Recovery	−.38	−.37	−.37	−.29	−.33	−.27	−.37	.55	.59		.59	.49	−.32	−.36	−.27	.75	.45	.74	.48
11 General Well-Being	−.56	−.49	−.59	−.25	−.25	−.34	−.34	.52	.80	.55		.49	−.30	−.41	−.27	.51	.31	.50	.28
12 Sleep Quality	−.70	−.64	−.60	−.43	−.41	−.46	−.63	.39	.54	.59	.62		−.17	−.38	−.37	.32	.13	.30	.15

Table 6.4a continued

Upper data matrix: A3

RESTQ Scales	1	2	3	4	5	6	7	8	9	10	11	12	13	14	15	16	17	18	19
13 Disturbed Breaks	–	–	–	–	–	–	–	–	–	–	–	–	–	.39	.34	–.29	–.29	–.31	–.32
14 Emotional Exhaustion	.49	.44	.43	.24	.36	.39	.58	–.23	–.16	–.26	–.22	–.39	–		.58	–.33	–.18	–.22	–.12
15 Injury	.13	.10	.16	.24	.22	.08	.31	.25	.04	.13	.05	.00	–	.41		–.23	–.04	–.08	.08
16 Being in Shape	–.39	–.22	–.26	–.14	–.27	–.23	–.36	.61	.43	.62	.48	.42	–	–.39	–.03		.61	.76	.65
17 Personal Accomplishment	–.40	–.22	–.26	–.16	–.28	–.35	–.31	.49	.44	.56	.44	.36	–	–.16	.26	.58		.57	.63
18 Self-Efficacy	–	–	–	–	–	–	–	–	–	–	–	–	–	–	–	–	–	–	.65
19 Self-Regulation	–.38	–.22	–.21	–.05	–.15	–.27	–.40	.61	.46	.57	.43	.44	–	–.32	.16	.71	–	–	

Lower data matrix: A2[1]

Note:
[1] In the prior version of the RESTQ-Sport, the development of the *Disturbed Breaks* and *Self-Efficacy* scales was not completed.

Table 6.4b Intercorrelation of the RESTQ-76 Sport Scales for the Canadian Samples C1 (n = 88) and C2 (n = 128)

RESTQ-Sport Scales								Upper data matrix: C1											
	1	2	3	4	5	6	7	8	9	10	11	12	13	14	15	16	17	18	19
1 General Stress		.75	.70	.69	.52	.68	.62	−.24	−.30	−.56	−.57	−.55	.48	.60	.46	−.44	−.26	−.43	−.15
2 Emotional Stress	.88		.83	.67	.54	.69	.69	−.23	−.30	−.58	−.59	−.59	.45	.53	.40	−.46	−.29	−.41	−.22
3 Social Stress	.80	.88		.64	.44	.57	.54	−.18	−.22	−.49	−.51	−.54	.50	.53	.45	−.40	−.28	−.36	−.16
4 Conflicts/ Pressure	.62	.72	.63		.56	.66	.51	−.14	−.24	−.47	−.49	−.58	.48	.51	.38	−.37	−.25	−.44	.01
5 Fatigue	.66	.73	.62	.65		.53	.61	−.05	−.27	−.49	−.41	−.58	.39	.33	.39	−.43	−.06	−.25	−.16
6 Lack of Energy	.69	.69	.65	.61	.62		.64	−.25	−.28	−.55	−.56	−.54	.39	.44	.46	−.42	−.19	−.37	−.21
7 Physical Complaints	.74	.78	.67	.63	.75	.73		−.21	−.36	−.54	−.57	−.59	.39	.49	.42	−.42	−.15	−.28	−.18
8 Success	.08	.18	.14	.26	.13	.02	.10		.62	.54	.53	.34	−.02	−.09	−.02	.45	.30	.31	.51
9 Social Recovery	−.13	−.08	−.09	.07	.05	.01	−.06	.57		.60	.78	.48	−.11	−.21	−.05	.62	.37	.36	.44
10 Physical Recovery	−.15	−.04	−.08	−.08	−.16	−.12	−.16	.66	.61		.80	.68	−.32	−.31	−.29	.75	.37	.54	.51
11 General Well-Being	−.29	−.23	−.24	−.08	−.12	−.05	−.15	.59	.82	.77		.71	−.30	−.41	−.21	.68	.41	.44	.44
12 Sleep Quality	−.17	−.19	−.11	−.27	−.34	−.14	−.23	.33	.32	.59	.53		−.46	−.48	−.24	.57	.27	.35	.32

(continued)

44

Table 6.4b   continued

Upper data matrix: C1

RESTQ-Sport Scales	1	2	3	4	5	6	7	8	9	10	11	12	13	14	15	16	17	18	19
13 Disturbed Breaks	.56	.60	.58	.50	.65	.55	.65	.12	.10	-.01	-.02	-.10		.58	.51	-.22	-.26	-.25	-.13
14 Emotional Exhaustion	.80	.77	.73	.61	.63	.63	.67	.09	-.16	-.09	-.23	-.09	65		.44	-.33	-.30	-.44	-.16
15 Injury	.52	.53	.42	.42	.53	.56	.66	.15	.13	-.01	.08	-.11	49	.49		-.31	.14	-.29	-.01
16 Being in Shape	-.14	-.08	.00	.02	-.11	-.13	-.18	.66	.61	.86	.68	.48	-.05	-.14	-.08		.58	.69	.60
17 Personal Accomplishment	-.06	.01	-.04	.02	.00	.07	.08	.56	.57	.64	.66	.45	.13	-.10	.13	.54		.73	.47
18 Self-Efficacy	-.17	-.09	-.08	.02	-.04	-.06	-.13	.60	.62	.75	.67	.35	.09	-.13	.02	.78	.65		.57
19 Self-Regulation	-.06	.03	.01	.04	.06	.00	.00	.57	.51	.65	.58	.36	.18	.00	.08	.69	.63	.77	

Lower data matrix: C2

Table 6.5 Intercorrelation of the RESTQ-76 Sport Scales for Females (*n* = 63) and Males (*n* = 65) for the Canadian Sample C2

Upper data matrix: C2 (female)

RESTQ-Sport Scales	1	2	3	4	5	6	7	8	9	10	11	12	13	14	15	16	17	18	19
1 General Stress		.92	.82	.68	.77	.70	.86	.18	.01	.04	-.10	-.03	.71	.82	.66	.03	.07	-.01	.12
2 Emotional Stress	.82		.88	.79	.80	.74	.88	.29	.08	.14	-.03	-.01	.74	.83	.61	.11	.17	.09	.24
3 Social Stress	.77	.89		.72	.67	.65	.76	.24	.03	.14	-.10	.05	.75	.77	.47	.17	.04	.04	.17
4 Conflicts/Pressure	.53	.61	.51		.71	.70	.71	.23	.07	.07	-.04	-.11	.63	.73	.37	.13	.02	.06	.18
5 Fatigue	.50	.63	.56	.57		.75	.83	.22	.22	.06	.06	-.13	.82	.73	.65	.05	.14	.12	.20
6 Lack of Energy	.69	.62	.65	.50	.46		.82	.10	.14	.08	.13	.03	.68	.67	.60	.03	.18	.06	.14
7 Physical Complaints	.58	.63	.54	.52	.66	.60		.19	.07	.10	.04	.02	.80	.81	.74	.03	.17	.07	.19
8 Success	-.11	-.02	-.01	.33	.00	-.07	.01		.64	.80	.64	.48	.27	.26	.23	.79	.69	.78	.81
9 Social Recovery	-.36	-.29	-.25	.07	-.16	-.11	-.19	.44		.70	.87	.48	.19	.06	.25	.69	.74	.72	.64
10 Physical Recovery	-.47	-.43	-.31	-.30	-.47	-.40	-.51	.40	.47		.81	.63	.14	.12	.15	.89	.81	.80	.72
11 General Well-Being	-.60	-.54	-.45	-.15	-.37	-.29	-.38	.51	.74	.71		.63	.11	.00	.22	.72	.84	.74	.67
12 Sleep Quality	-.38	-.44	-.32	-.47	-.60	-.33	-.51	.10	.10	.52	.39		.09	.06	.14	.55	.62	.48	.51

(continued)

Table 6.5 continued

RESTQ-Sport Scales		1	2	3	4	5	6	7	8	9	10	11	12	13	14	15	16	17	18	19
														Upper data matrix: C2 (female)						
13	Disturbed Breaks	.39	.39	.36	.33	.46	.36	.44	-.06	.03	-.22	-.17	-.31		.76	.63	.11	.14	.15	.23
14	Emotional Exhaustion	.78	.67	.68	.43	.49	.56	.49	-.19	-.46	-.40	-.57	-.27	.51		.64	.07	.05	.07	.23
15	Injury	.34	.43	.38	.50	.43	.48	.52	.11	.07	-.21	-.06	-.38	.29	.27		.05	.29	.17	.24
16	Being in Shape	-.43	-.38	-.27	-.10	-.35	-.34	-.46	.42	.45	.79	.61	.36	-.25	-.49	-.22		.69	.81	.73
17	Personal Accomplishment	-.26	-.21	-.16	.03	.17	-.06	-.02	.35	.32	.39	.39	.23	.15	-.29	-.02	.31		.75	.72
18	Self-Efficacy	-.38	-.33	-.21	-.04	-.24	-.18	-.34	.35	.49	.70	.58	.19	.04	-.37	-.11	.76	.52		.85
19	Self-Regulation	-.32	-.24	-.17	-.12	-.10	-.16	-.19	.21	.32	.55	.45	.19	.15	-.27	-.05	.62	.50	.67	
												Lower data matrix: C2 (male)								

47

Table 6.6 Intercorrelation of the RESTQ-76 Sport Scales for the German Sample R4 (*n* = 58) for the First and Second Surveys Over a 10-Day Period

Upper data matrix: R4 (first measurement)

RESTQ Scales	1	2	3	4	5	6	7	8	9	10	11	12	13	14	15	16	17	18	19
1 General Stress	.75	.63	.45	.35	.44	.66	.56	.12	-.48	-.57	-.55	-.49	.46	.70	.21	-.38	-.38	-.45	-.30
2 Emotional Stress			.60	.56	.25	.52	.45	.23	-.28	-.37	-.49	-.43	.38	.55	.23	-.23	-.09	-.32	-.13
3 Social Stress	.42	.72		.26	.18	.35	.30	.09	-.13	-.18	-.13	-.19	.24	.34	.29	-.11	-.02	-.12	-.13
4 Conflicts/Pressure	.25	.27	.18		.27	.28	.47	.60	.04	-.05	-.09	-.22	.31	.37	.15	.02	.23	.05	.29
5 Fatigue	.42	.32	.13	.44		.37	.55	.30	-.13	-.29	-.09	-.45	.56	.45	.47	-.34	.13	-.02	-.06
6 Lack of Energy	.60	.44	.09	.21	.57		.49	.01	-.08	-.27	-.03	-.34	.36	.56	.14	-.14	-.36	-.34	-.34
7 Physical Complaints	.40	.32	.07	.25	.64	.53		.41	-.25	-.39	-.29	-.36	.42	.50	.42	-.30	-.06	-.11	-.11
8 Success	-.02	.04	.13	.50	.18	.02	.03		.15	.09	.07	.03	.16	.09	-.01	.12	.54	.20	.44
9 Social Recovery	-.16	-.30	-.39	.18	.14	.00	-.07	.39		.66	.59	.41	-.21	-.17	-.11	.54	.40	.36	.41
10 Physical Recovery	-.43	-.39	-.20	-.04	-.20	-.30	-.36	.43	.56		.74	.67	-.40	-.25	-.18	.81	.48	.70	.57
11 General Well-Being	-.35	-.53	-.45	.03	.00	-.10	-.12	.39	.76	.73		.59	-.30	-.36	-.01	.60	.46	.72	.56
12 Sleep Quality	-.37	-.34	-.24	-.22	-.34	-.32	-.38	.02	.34	.54	.44		-.54	-.44	-.25	.72	.40	.56	.48

(continued)

Table 6.6   continued

Upper data matrix: R4 (first measurement)

RESTQ Scales	1	2	3	4	5	6	7	8	9	10	11	12	13	14	15	16	17	18	19
13 Disturbed Breaks	.39	.38	.23	.26	.44	.40	.43	.05	.09	-.12	.03	-.43		.39	.16	-.47	-.21	-.31	-.27
14 Emotional Exhaustion	.58	.41	.05	.40	.45	.48	.48	.16	.11	-.21	.03	-.39	.50		.41	-.24	-.31	-.30	-.20
15 Injury	.28	.22	.05	.41	.58	.44	.76	.18	.07	-.20	.02	-.29	.45	.37		-.17	.15	.12	.04
16 Being in Shape	-.41	-.41	-.21	-.14	-.42	-.38	-.43	.28	.47	.77	.60	.71	-.48	-.36	-.35		.50	.68	.57
17 Personal Accomplishment	-.35	-.35	-.18	.11	-.03	-.11	-.16	.42	.42	.50	.51	.33	-.14	-.26	.06	.52		.68	.70
18 Self-Efficacy	-.41	-.45	-.27	-.01	-.12	-.24	-.20	.41	.51	.68	.59	.42	-.27	-.37	.00	.66	.68		.72
19 Self-Regulation	-.32	-.31	-.13	.21	.01	-.24	-.21	.48	.40	.53	.42	.42	-.35	-.41	.00	.60	.62	.73	

Lower data matrix: R4 (second measurement)

Table 6.7a Two-Factor-Solution (With a >.25) for the General Scales of the RESTQ-85 Sport for the American Sample A3 ($n = 77$)

	RESTQ-Sport scales	Factor 1	Factor 2	h^2
1	General Stress	.81	−.33	.77
2	Emotional Stress	.82	—	.70
3	Social Stress	.73	—	.58
4	Conflicts/Pressure	.80	—	.66
5	Fatigue	.68	—	.52
6	Lack of Energy	.68	−.26	.53
7	Physical Complaints	.73	−.35	.65
8	Success	—	.81	.68
9	Social Recovery	−.31	.69	.54
10	Physical Recovery	−.34	.74	.67
11	General Well-Being	−.52	.67	.72
12	Sleep Quality	−.58	.42	.51
	Eigenvalue	5.97	1.56	
	Variance in %	49.7	13.0	

Table 6.7b Two-Factor-Solution (With a >.25) for the General Scales of the RESTQ-80 Sport for the Canadian Sample C1 ($n = 88$)

	RESTQ scales	Factor 1	Factor 2	h^2
1	General Stress	.83	—	.73
2	Emotional Stress	.87	—	.80
3	Social Stress	.81	—	.67
4	Conflicts/Pressure	.81	—	.67
5	Fatigue	.72	—	.53
6	Lack of Energy	.78	—	.66
7	Physical Complaints	.75	−.28	.64
8	Success	—	.83	.68
9	Social Recovery	—	.88	.80
10	Physical Recovery	−.51	.70	.77
11	General Well-Being	−.51	.77	.85
12	Sleep Quality	−.62	.49	.64
	Eigenvalue	6.72	1.71	
	Variance in %	56.0	14.3	

Table 6.7c   Two-Factor-Solution (With a >.25) for the General Scales of the RESTQ-76 Sport for the Canadian Sample C2 (n = 128)

	RESTQ-Sport scales	Factor 1	Factor 2	h^2
1	General Stress	.89	—	.80
2	Emotional Stress	.94	—	.89
3	Social Stress	.87	—	.75
4	Conflicts/Pressure	.81	—	.66
5	Fatigue	.83	—	.70
6	Lack of Energy	.81	—	.66
7	Physical Complaints	.87	—	.76
8	Success	—	.79	.67
9	Social Recovery	—	.83	.69
10	Physical Recovery	—	.89	.80
11	General Well-Being	—	.91	.86
12	Sleep Quality	—	.63	.45
Eigenvalue		5.43	3.27	
Variance in %		45.3	27.2	

Table 6.8a   Two-Factor-Solution (With a >.25) for the Sport-Specific Scales of the RESTQ-85 Sport for the American Sample A3 (n = 77)

	RESTQ scales	Factor 1	Factor 2	h^2
13	Disturbed Breaks	−.30	.59	.44
14	Emotional Exhaustion	—	.84	.73
15	Injury	—	.88	.78
16	Being in Shape	.84	−.28	.80
17	Personal Accomplishment	.81	—	.66
18	Self-Efficacy	.86	—	.75
19	Self-Regulation	.88	—	.77
Eigenvalue		3.26	1.65	
Variance in %		46.6	23.5	

Table 6.8b Two-Factor-Solution (With a >.25) for the Sport-Specific Scales of the RESTQ-80 Sport for the Canadian Sample C1 (n = 88)

	RESTQ-Sport scales	Factor 1	Factor 2	h^2
13	Disturbed Breaks	—	.84	.71
14	Emotional Exhaustion	—	.78	.67
15	Injury	—	.80	.64
16	Being in Shape	.82	—	.73
17	Personal Accomplishment	.81	—	.68
18	Self-Efficacy	.86	—	.81
19	Self-Regulation	.81	—	.67
	Eigenvalue	3.36	1.54	
	Variance in %	48.0	22.1	

Table 6.8c Two-Factor-Solution (With a >.25) for the Sport-Specific Scales of the RESTQ-76 Sport for the Canadian Sample C2 (n = 128)

	RESTQ-Sport scales	Factor 1	Factor 2	h^2
13	Disturbed Breaks	—	.87	.76
14	Emotional Exhaustion	—	.86	.75
15	Injury	—	.77	.60
16	Being in Shape	.87	—	.77
17	Personal Accomplishment	.80	—	.65
18	Self-Efficacy	.92	—	.85
19	Self-Regulation	.89	—	.80
	Eigenvalue	3.06	2.12	
	Variance in %	43.7	30.3	

Table 6.9 Correlation Between the Multidimensional Physical Symptom List (MPSL) and the RESTQ-Sport for the German Sample R2 ($n = 42$)

Scales of the Multidimensional Physical Symptom List

RESTQ-Sport Scales	MPSL 1	MPSL 2	MPSL 3	MPSL 4	MPSL 5	MPSL 6	MPSL 7	MPSL 8	MPSL 9
1 General Stress	.30	.52	.36	.53	.29	.13	.24	.05	.40
2 Emotional Stress	.41	.45	.13	.43	.09	.28	.05	.28	.31
3 Social Stress	.22	.27	.06	.25	−.14	.25	−.04	.21	.17
4 Conflicts/Pressure	.27	.30	.17	.31	.13	.19	.17	.16	.18
5 Fatigue	.39	.33	.14	.35	.14	.30	−.01	.49	.45
6 Lack of Energy	.39	.53	.22	.44	.35	.24	.08	.24	.47
7 Physical Complaints	.45	.65	.49	.48	.46	.31	.20	.24	.78
8 Success	.08	.13	.14	.00	.04	−.16	.06	.08	−.11
9 Social Recovery	−.20	−.02	.11	.10	−.01	−.04	.10	−.20	−.02
10 Physical Recovery	−.33	−.48	−.30	−.46	−.16	−.36	−.26	−.07	−.57
11 General Well-Being	−.16	−.05	.11	−.14	.01	−.19	.07	−.18	−.12
12 Sleep Quality	−.28	−.36	−.25	−.45	−.13	−.48	−.29	.11	−.33
13 Disturbed Breaks	.31	.56	.33	.41	.25	.12	.18	.19	.47
14 Emotional Exhaustion	.39	.54	.40	.45	.38	.10	.29	.13	.44
15 Injury	.48	.63	.44	.43	.48	.25	.06	.29	.79
16 Being in Shape	−.24	−.36	−.20	−.41	−.18	−.21	−.12	−.12	−.50
17 Personal Accomplishment	.15	.16	.22	.00	.16	−.23	.17	−.08	.13
18 Self-Efficacy	−.18	−.32	−.13	−.36	−.21	−.25	−.14	.01	−.37
19 Self-Regulation	−.17	−.25	−.13	−.30	−.17	−.25	−.16	.00	−.33

MPSL 1 = Circulation (central)
MPSL 2 = Respiration (stressed)
MPSL 3 = Circulation (peripheral)
MPSL 4 = Muscle System
MPSL 5 = Stomach-Intestinal System
MPSL 6 = Thermoregulation-Heat Reduction
MPSL 7 = Thermoregulation-Heat Storage
MPSL 8 = Appetite
MPSL 9 = General Physical Oversensitivity

Table 6.10   Correlation Between the RESTQ-Sport and the POMS for the Canadian Sample C1 ($n = 65$)

	RESTQ-Sport scales	Scales of the Profile of Mood States					
		Tension	Depression	Anger	Vigor	Fatigue	Confusion
1	General Stress	.70	.74	.73	−.19	.45	.72
2	Emotional Stress	.75	.61	.65	−.34	.51	.64
3	Social Stress	.75	.69	.75	−.34	.50	.71
4	Conflicts/Pressure	.68	.55	.46	−.30	.45	.67
5	Fatigue	.40	.34	.28	−.20	.50	.33
6	Lack of Energy	.59	.45	.43	−.38	.57	.69
7	Physical Complaints	.42	.48	.46	−.29	.55	.38
8	Success	−.14	−.16	−.13	.37	−.09	−.19
9	Social Recovery	−.32	−.33	−.17	.44	−.28	−.24
10	Physical Recovery	−.57	−.42	−.43	.49	−.50	−.46
11	General Well-Being	−.62	−.47	−.46	.60	−.52	−.51
12	Sleep Quality	−.67	−.45	−.49	.45	−.58	−.56
13	Disturbed Breaks	.51	.38	.40	−.28	.42	.45
14	Emotional Exhaustion	.50	.58	.50	−.31	.42	.56
15	Injury	.38	.43	.35	−.23	.56	.39
16	Being in Shape	−.38	−.34	−.25	.61	−.49	−.34
17	Personal Accomplishment	−.25	−.22	−.13	.29	−.18	−.12
18	Self-Efficacy	−.34	−.40	−.22	.40	−.27	−.36
19	Self-Regulation	−.10	−.10	−.13	.43	−.20	−.05

Table 6.11 Correlation Between the State-Trait Anxiety Inventory and the RESTQ-Sport for the American Samples A1 ($n = 33$) and A2 ($n = 84$)

RESTQ-Sport Scales/measurement	State form[1]					Trait form		A2[2]
	A1 1	A1 2	A1 3	A1 4	A1 5	A1 1	A1 4	1
1 General Stress	.63	.65	.75	.53	.78	.65	.70	.63
2 Emotional Stress	.35	.62	.58	.33	.65	.38	.55	.53
3 Social Stress	.57	.71	.56	.44	.68	.59	.65	.47
4 Conflicts/Pressure	.41	.65	.53	.41	.40	.49	.60	.39
5 Fatigue	.26	.35	.38	.13	.61	.42	.36	.42
6 Lack of Energy	.43	.62	.68	.23	.57	.62	.47	.54
7 Physical Complaints	.46	.46	.64	.44	.65	.58	.60	.39
8 Success	−.28	−.47	−.58	−.50	−.37	−.26	−.45	−.38
9 Social Recovery	−.55	−.46	−.61	−.43	−.51	−.47	−.50	−.46
10 Physical Recovery	−.33	−.41	−.56	−.56	−.60	−.37	−.63	−.48
11 General Well-Being	−.56	−.66	−.80	−.77	−.67	−.70	−.72	−.59
12 Sleep Quality	—	—	—	—	—	—	—	−.56
13 Disturbed Breaks	—	—	—	—	—	—	—	—
14 Emotional Exhaustion	—	—	—	—	—	—	—	.33
15 Injury	—	—	—	—	—	—	—	−.01
16 Being in Shape	—	—	—	—	—	—	—	−.39
17 Personal Accomplishment	—	—	—	—	—	—	—	−.42
18 Self-Efficacy	—	—	—	—	—	—	—	—
19 Self-Regulation	—	—	—	—	—	—	—	−.28

Note:
[1]Correlations between the RESTQ and state form of the STAI for five measurements and for the trait form for two measurements, respectively. In the prior version of the RESTQ, the development of the *Sleep Quality* scale was not completed.
[2]In the prior version of the RESTQ-Sport, the development of the *Disturbed Breaks* and *Self-Efficacy* scales was not completed.

Table 6.12 Correlation Between the Volitional Component Questionnaire (VCQ) and the RESTQ-Sport for the German Sample G1 ($n = 71$)

RESTQ-Sport scales	Scales of the Volitional Component Questionnaire											
	VCQ 1	VCQ 2	VCQ 3	VCQ 4	VCQ 5	VCQ 6	VCQ 7	VCQ 8	VCQ 9	VCQ 10	VCQ 11	VCQ 12
1 General Stress	−.29	−.40	−.46	-.43	−.32	−.48	.27	.45	.49	.46	.47	.39
2 Emotional Stress	-.32	−.43	−.31	−.33	−.35	−.38	.27	.46	.36	.37	.32	.20
3 Social Stress	−.27	−.26	−.10	−.28	−.30	−.31	−.34	.53	.34	.24	.31	.25
4 Conflicts/ Pressure	−.08	−.08	−.11	−.20	−.19	−.13	.25	.41	.25	.33	.23	.34
5 Fatigue	.00	−.10	−.13	−.24	−.14	−.08	.30	.23	.13	.08	.00	.30
6 Lack of Energy	−.23	−.26	−.28	−.30	−.43	−.22	.49	.43	.17	.10	.14	.46
7 Physical Complaints	−.13	−.18	−.20	−.33	−.27	−.23	.42	.25	.18	.16	.19	.20
8 Success	.31	.42	.35	.29	.27	.32	−.01	−.21	−.22	−.14	−.19	−.02
9 Social Recovery	.36	.37	.44	.29	.14	.30	−.09	−.19	−.23	−.16	−.26	−.12
10 Physical Recovery	.45	.55	.54	.48	.50	.48	−.19	−.25	−.23	−.10	−.13	−.07
11 General Well-Being	.46	.57	.65	.49	.36	.51	−.05	−.32	−.36	−.25	−.29	−.17
12 Sleep Quality	.29	.34	.44	.45	.37	.33	−.24	−.36	−.35	−.25	−.30	−.26
13 Disturbed Breaks	−.11	−.07	−.12	−.27	−.15	−.23	.42	.30	.16	.09	.12	.44
14 Emotional Exhaustion	−.04	−.13	−.09	−.26	−.12	−.29	.18	−.01	.29	.25	.32	.15
15 Injury	−.05	−.11	−.04	−.22	−.35	−.25	.44	.22	.12	.13	.17	.20
16 Being in Shape	.39	.51	.50	.54	.52	.52	−.22	−.32	−.29	−.23	−.26	−.15
17 Personal Accomplishment	.41	.36	.39	.39	.43	.33	−.28	−.37	−.18	−.05	−.17	−.04
18 Self-Efficacy	.42	.63	.63	.55	.57	.56	−.28	−.41	−.34	−.32	−.35	−.24
19 Self-Regulation	.42	.55	.55	.50	.45	.43	−.18	−.29	−.30	−.29	−.32	−.13

VCQ 1 = Self-Determination
VCQ 2 = Positive Self-Motivation
VCQ 3 = Emotion Control
VCQ 4 = Self-Relaxation

VCQ 5 = Initiative
VCQ 6 = Volitional Self-Efficacy
VCQ 7 = Procrastination
VCQ 8 = Susceptibility to Intrusions

VCQ 9 = Alienation
VCQ 10 = Rumination
VCQ 11 = Passive Avoidance
VCQ 12 = Self-Discipline

overall scores can be developed from the positive correlations within the stress and recovery scales. To get a closer look at the empirical distribution of the possible recovery-stress state patterns, the group is divided at the median of the recovery and stress area and the parts are compared with each other. In the analysis of the four recovery-stress state patterns *(I. low stress - low recovery, II. high stress - low recovery, III. low stress - high recovery, IV. high stress - high recovery)*, a consistent distribution pattern has been found across different samples (table 6.13).

The recovery-stress patterns *II. high stress - low recovery* and *III. low stress - high recovery* each represent about one-third of the empirical distribution. The other third is shared by the patterns *I. low stress - low recovery* and *IV. high stress - high recovery*. As shown in table 6.13, the exact distribution of the four types varies slightly within the different analysis samples, although it remains remarkably constant as a whole.

For the German sample G1, a two-factor multivariate analysis of variance was utilized to show the differences in the habitual components of volitional control between the recovery-stress state patterns. Due to the sufficient distribution of the scale values from the psychometric tested questionnaire, it is apparent that the estimation of the multivariate effects after Hotelling (Bortz, 1993) is adequately robust for the data at hand. The 2×2 univariate analysis of variance came up with follow-up tests for every scale (table 6.14).

The 2×2 analyses did not show significant interaction, but only the main effects of recovery and stress. The main effect for recovery is highly significant for the habitual components of volitional control ($F(12,61) = 5.53; p < .001$), and the main effect for stress is also significant ($F(12,61) = 2.13; p < .05$). Relevant for the factor stress are the univariate follow-up tests for the scales *Procrastination* and *Self-Discipline*. These scales are not significant in the

follow-up tests for recovery, as are the scales *Susceptibility to Intrusions* and *Alienation*. All of the other VCQ scales reach a minimum significance level of *p* < .05. The analyses show that the difference between most motivational components of the VCQ can be reduced to the factor recovery. The scales *Procrastination, Susceptibility to Intrusions, Alienation,* and *Self-Discipline* do not fit into this pattern (see also Beckmann & Kellmann, 2001).

Changes in the Recovery-Stress State

The recovery-stress state is dependent on current activities regarding stress and recovery. Although the recovery-stress state is stable in the face of temporary functional fluctuations, it is affected by activities in the daily life of individuals. For example, vacations or training load changes influence the recovery-stress state quite a bit.

Effects of Vacation

In a repeated measurement study, Kellmann, Johnson, and Wrisberg (1998) found significant improvement of the recovery-stress state in American female swimmers (NCAA Division I) after a four-day Thanksgiving break. Twenty-one athletes (age *M*: 19.43 years; *SD*: 1.25) completed the RESTQ-Sport and the POMS (McNair et al., 1992) throughout the season. The swimmers were instructed to complete the questionnaires 48 hours before each intercollegiate competition. The first competition took place six days prior to the four-day Thanksgiving break. The second took place two days after the holidays. The analysis with paired *t*-tests showed a dramatic improvement in the recovery-stress state after the four-day vacation (figure 6.1). The general stress level diminished and recovery increased over the vacation break, especially *Physical Recovery*,

Table 6.13   Empirical Distribution of Recovery-Stress State Patterns for American (A2, A3), Canadian (C1, C2), and German (R4) Samples

Recovery-stress states	A2 $n = 91$	A3 $n = 86$	C1 $n = 85$	C2 $n = 128$	R4 $n = 58$	Mean
I. low stress - low recovery	16.5%	17.4%	15.3%	15.6%	24.1%	**17.8%**
II. high stress - low recovery	34.1%	33.7%	34.1%	33.6%	31.0%	**33.3%**
III. low stress - high recovery	31.9%	34.9%	31.8%	33.6%	29.3%	**32.3%**
IV. high stress - high recovery	17.5%	14.0%	18.8%	17.2%	15.6%	**16.6%**

Table 6.14   Two-Factor Multivariate Analysis of Variance of the VCQ and the Recovery-Stress States for the German Sample G1 ($n = 76$)

VCQ scales	Pattern I M	Pattern I SD	Pattern II M	Pattern II SD	Pattern III M	Pattern III SD	Pattern IV M	Pattern IV SD	$p(R)$ df (1,72)	$p(S)$ df (1,72)	$p(RxS)$ df (1,72)
	$n = 12$		$n = 25$		$n = 29$		$n = 10$				
1 Self-Determination	1.55	.46	1.69	.57	2.07	.49	1.96	.51	.004	.912	.350
2 Positive Self-Motivation	1.28	.64	1.33	.43	1.95	.40	1.80	.37	.000	.663	.411
3 Emotional Control	1.05	.53	1.22	.50	1.88	.45	1.78	.56	.000	.802	.288
4 Self-Relaxation	1.33	.45	1.23	.52	1.81	.57	1.52	.38	.005	.142	.480
5 Initiative	1.50	.46	1.42	.44	1.90	.59	1.76	.51	.006	.403	.797
6 Volitional Self-Efficacy	1.68	.46	1.78	.54	2.41	.39	2.24	.40	.000	.750	.267
7 Procrastination	.62	.37	1.22	.60	.90	.59	1.30	.37	.184	.001	.465
8 Susceptibility to Intrusions	1.12	.57	1.42	.65	.90	.61	1.08	.47	.074	.120	.707
9 Alienation	1.08	.45	1.20	.50	.86	.41	1.14	.59	.239	.100	.498
10 Rumination	1.03	.78	1.38	.61	.81	.57	.98	.27	.045	.096	.561
11 Passive Avoidance	.83	.61	1.06	.56	.57	.50	.76	.46	.044	.135	.897
12 Self-Discipline	1.33	.48	1.65	.38	1.28	.57	1.50	.47	.426	.035	.695

Recovery-stress state patterns:
   I.   low stress - low recovery
   II. high stress - low recovery
   III. low stress - high recovery
   IV. high stress - high recovery

General Well-Being, and *Sleep Quality.* Matching those changes, the sport-specific scales *Injury, Emotional Exhaustion,* and *Disturbed Breaks* decreased.

This result is not surprising, since *taking a break* is the purpose of a vacation; however, it is also important to look at individual situations. Athletes who had to travel a long distance to get home could not profit from the break as much as swimmers who lived near the university. For some, Thanksgiving vacation was a time to rest and enjoy a slower pace of life. For others, it was characterized by higher emotional intensity associated with activities involving family, friends, and significant others. Although such activities may represent a change in the normal training regimen, they may not be less emotionally stressful.

For a detailed analysis, the individual interpretation of the RESTQ-Sport is useful, because it gives the support staff (e.g., coach, sport psychologist) a clear picture of the athlete's recovery-stress state.

The study made clear that recovery should not only be understood as an integral part of training, but should also be recognized in activities apart from sport that affect the athlete's recovery-stress state.

Effects Within a Training Camp

Since 1994, each year during the training camp for the World Championships, members of the German Junior National Rowing Team have been monitored psychologically with the RESTQ-Sport (Kellmann, Kallus, Steinacker, & Lormes, 1997; Kellmann et al., 2001; Kellmann, Kallus, Günther et al., 1997). During the camp (and before the Championships), the athletes completed the RESTQ-Sport up to eight times within a six-week period. In parallel with the questionnaire measurements, the athletes underwent a sport medical assessment (i.e., lactate, creatine kinase, urea, uric acid).

This interdisciplinary approach helps coaches, physicians, and sport psychologists share informa-

RESTQ-76 Sport Profile:

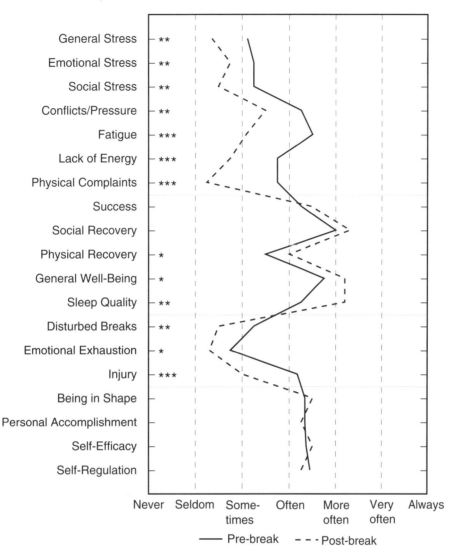

Figure 6.1   Recovery-stress states of American female swimmers (A4) before and after the Thanksgiving vacation [p-value: *: $.05 \geq p > .01$; **: $.01 \geq p > .001$; ***: $p < .001$].

tion and draw mutual conclusions. One goal is to identify recovery-stress states of athletes that deviate from individual or group profiles (see chapter 3). To integrate the sport psychologist into the team of coaches and athletes, his/her immediate feedback on the RESTQ results is needed. Questionnaires can give coaches and physicians the fast feedback needed for immediate interventions.

Several studies (Ferger, 1998a, 1998b; Kellmann et al., 1997; Kellmann & Günther, 2000) have shown that the RESTQ-Sport assesses physical and psychological stress over different training phases, which means that the recovery-stress state reflects the training load. Using the RESTQ-Sport, Kellmann and Günther (2000) investigated changes in stress and recovery in rowers during preparation for the

1996 Atlanta Olympic Games. The results show that a *dose-response relationship* exists between training volume indicated by the average number of minutes of daily extensive endurance training and the subjective assessment of stress and recovery. High training load is indicated by an elevated level of stress and, at the same time, a decreased level of recovery. This supports the findings of Kellmann et al. (1997), who chose the average number of daily rowed kilometers as an indicator for training volume. In their study, participants completed the RESTQ-Sport five times during training camp and before the Junior World Championships in Rowing (T1: on arrival at training camp; T2-T4: during training camp; T5: before preliminaries). All athletes were supervised by coaches of the German Rowing

Association, who determined the training schedule. Figure 6.2 displays the relationship between the average number of kilometers rowed each day and the consequences illustrated by the scale *Lack of Energy*.

Figure 6.2 reveals the development of the relationship between rowed kilometers and the scores in *Lack of Energy* during training camp. These results were not surprising and reflect the training schedule. They indicate the validity of the RESTQ-Sport for monitoring training.

Even more complex presentations of training volume and intensity (Kellmann et al., 2001; Steinacker, Lormes, Lehmann, & Altenburg, 1998) reveal the dose-response relationship described above. In addition, the same relationship between training load and the RESTQ-Sport has been found for soccer (Ferger, 1998a, 1998b; Hogg, 2000), basketball (Jochum, 1994), and mountain biking (Kallus & Kellmann, 2000).

As figure 6.3 illustrates, the RESTQ-Sport data can also be used to evaluate the training schedule after the season (Kellmann & Altenburg, 2000). Did the training schedule have the desired effects on the athletes? Over several years, RESTQ-Sport data could provide feedback and show whether the training effects actually went in the desired direction.

Figure 6.3 shows the change in male rowers in the *Fitness/Being in Shape* scale during training camp over three years. As can be seen, the training schedule was modified over the years, and one purpose of the 1998 training camp was to start with high-impact weight lifting training.

Relationship to Physiological/ Medical Data

Steinacker et al. (1999, 2000) reported on the time characteristics of hormones and the course of RESTQ-Sport results. *Physical Complaints*, as reported in the RESTQ-Sport, are highest during the phase of most intensive training, which correlates with increased cortisol and creatine kinase (CK). If *Physical Complaints* decrease, the distribution of cortisol and CK also declines. In the same way, the peak amount of norepinephrine corresponds to *Fatigue*. The authors suggested that multivariable analysis should be used in future research, considering physiological and psychological parameters in different courses of time.

Steinacker et al. (1999) also noted that during training camp, the reported illnesses reached their peak with the most reported *Physical Complaints*. The sample R^2 was analyzed to clarify this correla-

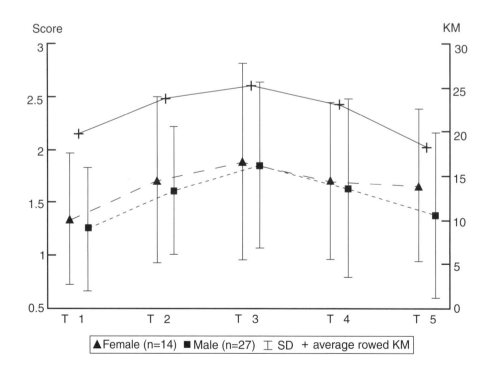

Figure 6.2   Arithmetic mean and standard deviation (SD) of the RESTQ-Sport *Lack of Energy* scale over five measurements (T1-T5), as well as the mean daily rowing kilometers (KM) for the preceding three days.

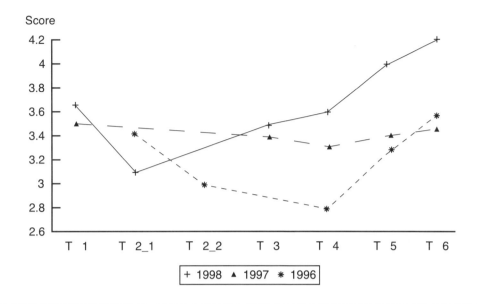

Figure 6.3 Arithmetic mean of the RESTQ-Sport *Fitness/Being in Shape* scale over three years for male rowers during the training camp before the Junior World Championships in Rowing. Whereas five measurements were taken in 1996 (T2_1, T2_2, T4, T5, T6) and 1997 (T1, T3, T4, T5, T6), six were used in 1998 (T1, T2_1, T3, T4, T5, T6). To compare the data, the assessments were adapted to the time schedule that describes the development over three years.

tion and to verify whether, using the RESTQ-Sport, a prediction can be made about an athlete's forthcoming medical examination. The following criteria were valid for the analysis:

- Reported recently sick are those athletes who did not have a doctor's appointment three days prior to filling out the RESTQ-Sport. The reason behind this somewhat conservative decision was that persons with acute complaints will express these in the RESTQ-Sport. Therefore, the verification of predicted effects was related to medically inconspicuous athletes.

- All forms of treatment were weighed equally; that is, no differentiation was made between a cold, muscle tension, or other complaints.

- The analysis of reported sickness applies to the day of the survey and the following two days, because the RESTQ-Sport has proven to have a high test-retest reliability for the duration of two days, and this time frame is considered to be stable.

In the analysis, the group of athletes who recently reported being sick (newly sick) were compared with the remaining athletes (rest group). Every RESTQ-Sport scale was divided at the paramedian. The evaluation of the accomplishments was organized with a four-field table using a Chi^2-test. At the time periods T1, T2, and T3, some scales reached a significant Chi^2-value ($p < .05$), whereas at T4 and T5,

consistent patterns were present. At time T4, the distribution of the physically oriented scales (*Physical Complaints, Physical Recovery, Being in Shape, Injury*), *Self-Regulation* and *Self-Efficacy* had a significant systematic relationship. The athletes who consider themselves to be highly stressed and/or insufficiently recovered will probably go to the doctor within the next two days. This becomes apparent in the distribution of the *Injury* scale, which is shown in table 6.15.

At time T4, there is still no significant distribution of the *Personal Accomplishment* scale (table 6.15). Just before the World Championships, the distribution of the *Personal Accomplishment* scale changes dramatically (table 6.16).

Eleven of the 14 athletes showing low values for *Personal Accomplishment* consulted their team doctor. In the RESTQ-Sport, significant distribution patterns were also present in the general recovery area (*Social Recovery, Physical Recovery, General Well-Being*), and a trend was found for the *General Stress* and *Emotional Stress* scales. The distributions for *Fatigue, Self-Efficacy,* and *Self-Regulation* remained stable.

A change in the meaning of the physically oriented areas just before competition seems to be portrayed by the distribution patterns, especially their changes in time periods T4 and T5. After a long preparation period, the various aspects of recovery, as well as *Personal Accomplishment, Self-Efficacy,* and *Self-Regulation*, become increasingly important as the competition gets closer.

Table 6.15   Four-Field Table of the Acute Notifications of Sickness and the RESTQ-Sport *Injury* and *Personal Accomplishment* Scales at Time T4

	Injury				Personal Accomplishment		
	Low	**High**	**Σ**		**Low**	**High**	**Σ**
New sick reports	1	11	12	New sick reports	8	4	12
Rest group	19	11	30	Rest group	16	14	30
Σ	20	22	42	Σ	24	18	42

Chi^2– value: 10.4; df: 1; p = .001   Chi^2– value: .62; df: 1; p = .43

Table 6.16   Four-Field Table of the Acute Notifications of Sickness and the RESTQ-Sport *Personal Accomplishment* Scale at T5

			Personal Accomplishment		
			Low	**High**	**Σ**
	New sick reports		11	3	14
	Rest group		9	18	27
	Σ		20	21	41

Chi^2– value: 7.55; df: 1; p = .006

Performance Prediction by the RESTQ-Sport

Kellmann and Kallus (1993) presented the option of using the RESTQ-Sport to predict performance prior to competition. To replicate those findings, Kellmann, Kallus, and Kurz (1996) used the same procedure in the following analysis. The results confirm a close relationship between the recovery-stress state and performance in competition for the general stress-oriented and the recovery-related areas, as well as for most single scales. In the present context, the results for the *Disturbed Breaks* scale are described (table 6.17). For a complete description of the procedure for the 3 × 3 field-contingency table and the use of placement as an outcome measure, see Kellmann (1991), Kellmann and Kallus (1993), and Kurz (1995).

In general, athletes who describe themselves as *highly disturbed* during breaks finish in lower places (5th and 6th place) during competition. Simultaneously, not all athletes who report being *minimally disturbed* necessarily finish first in competition, which underlines the complex interaction between stress and recovery.

To specifically examine the results of table 6.17, the extreme groups, *minimally disturbed* and *highly disturbed*, were analyzed. In this step, the first through fourth places were categorized into one group (1st-4th place vs. 5th-6th place, table 6.18). Those athletes who scored moderately in *Disturbed Breaks* were excluded from the analysis. In earlier studies, it became obvious that the RESTQ-Sport can mainly predict athletes who finish in lower places in competition (Kellmann, 1991; Kellmann & Kallus, 1993). A clear differentiation between 1st place and 2nd through 4th place turned out to be more difficult. Therefore, those categories were summarized. Because of the low sample size, the Fisher-Yates test was performed for an exact analysis of the 2 × 2 table (Lienert, 1973).

Based on this procedure, a clear relationship (p < .05) was revealed between the extent of *Disturbed Breaks* and performance in competition. Athletes who scored as *highly disturbed* during breaks on the questionnaire have a greater chance of finishing last in competition, whereas *minimally disturbed* athletes have a greater chance of finishing up front (1st-4th place).

| Table 6.17 | 3 × 3 Field-Contingency Table for *Disturbed Breaks* from the RESTQ-Sport and the Ability Groups (Places 1, 2-4, 5-6) at the Preliminaries of the 1993 German Swimming Team Competition (*n* = 26) |

| | | Place | | | |
		1	**2,3,4**	**5,6**	**Total**
	Minimally disturbed	2	6	1	9
Disturbed	Partially disturbed	2	2	4	8
Breaks	Highly disturbed	2	0	7	9
	Total	6	8	12	26

Chi^2 – value: 11.01; df: 4; p = .026

| Table 6.18 | Extreme Group Analysis According to the Four-Field Table for *Disturbed Breaks* of the RESTQ-Sport and the Ability Groups (Places 1-4, 5-6) at the Preliminaries of the 1993 German Swimming Team Competition. Subsample (*n* = 18); eight athletes with medium stress scores are excluded (see table 6.17) |

| | | Place | | |
		1-4	**5,6**	**Total**
	Minimally disturbed	8	1	9
Disturbed	Highly disturbed	2	7	9
Breaks	Total	10	8	18

Fisher-Yates test for the exact probabilities (two-tailed): p = .0152.

Summary

- The RESTQ-Sport has proven to be reliable and valid.

- The results of the RESTQ-Sport are stable in the face of short-term functionary fluctuations and short-term changes in recovery-stress state.

- The different stress scales as well as the different recovery scales correlate positively with the scales of the related areas; however, they have a moderate negative relationship with the scales of the opposite areas.

- All factor analyses clearly suggest one stress-related and one recovery-related factor for the general as well as for the sport-specific parts of the RESTQ-Sport.

- The Profile of Mood States *Tension*, *Depression*, *Anger*, *Fatigue*, and *Confusion* scales are negatively correlated with recovery-related scales, whereas the *Vigor* scale shows a positive relationship. The opposite is true for the stress-related scales.

- Positive correlations exist between stress and anxiety of the State-Trait Anxiety Inventory, and negative correlations exist between anxiety and recovery.

- The recovery-stress patterns *II. high stress - low recovery* and *III. low stress - high recovery* each make up approximately one-third of the empirical distribution. The other third is shared by the patterns *I. low stress - low recovery* and *IV. high stress - high recovery*.

- Motivational components interact with the recovery-stress state.

- The recovery-stress state reflects the training load.

- The RESTQ-Sport also makes it possible to observe individuals and/or groups over the course of a season, during training camps, as well as over many years.

- Corresponding changes with training volume exist between hormone levels and RESTQ-Sport results.

- A close relationship exists between the recovery-stress state and performance in competition.

Summary of the RESTQ-Sport Features

The RESTQ-Sport provides coaches, sport psychologists, and athletes with important information for use during the training process. For other members of the supporting staff, such as trainers, physio- and massage therapists, physiologists, or medical doctors, the RESTQ-Sport also helps in understanding the current recovery-stress state of athletes. Of course, this information is also relevant if coaches and athletes have not been in contact with each other for a longer time period (e.g., because of vacation or injuries).

To adequately manage the training process and prevent overtraining, it is important to gain information about the athlete's state in the past few days. Moreover, information based on an athlete's subjective perception is helpful for the coaching staff because the coaches' and athlete's perceptions often differ. By using the RESTQ-Sport, athletes and coaches can be informed about the importance of some daily activities. It can demonstrate how these activities relate to stress/recovery, as well as their effects on performance in athletics.

The RESTQ-Sport also makes it possible to observe individuals and/or groups over an entire season (Ferger, 1998a, 1998b), during training camps (Hogg, 2000; Kellmann et al., 2001; Kellmann & Günther, 1999, 2000), and also over many years (Kellmann & Altenburg, 2000). Due to the sufficient temporary stability of the results, the assessment can be done up to 48 hours before competition, allowing enough time for coaches or sport psychologists to intervene and optimize the recovery-stress state. During performance plateaus (times when performance does not increase), a survey may also be beneficial to athletes and coaches in determining whether the intensity of training should be increased or decreased.

References

Allmer, H. (1996). *Erholung und Gesundheit: Grundlagen, Ergebnisse und Maßnahmen* [Recovery and Health: Basics, Results and Interventions]. Göttingen: Hogrefe.

Allmer, H., & Niehues, C. (1989). Individuelle Erholungsmaßnahmen nach mentalen Arbeitsanforderungen unter Berücksichtigung der sportlichen Aktivität [Individual Recovery After Mental Workload While Considering the Physical Activity]. *Brennpunkt der Sportwissenschaft, 3*, 164-183.

Anshel, M.H. (1997). *Sport Psychology: From Theory to Practice*. Scottsdale, AZ: Gorsuch Scaribrick.

Bandura, A. (1977). Self-Efficacy: Toward a Unifying Theory of Behavioral Change. *Psychological Review, 84*, 191-215.

Beckmann, J., & Kellmann, M. (2001). Self-regulation and Recovery. Manuscript submitted for publication.

Berger, B.G., Motl, R.W., Butki, B.D., Martin, D.T., Wilkinson, J.G., & Owen, D.R. (1999). Mood and Cycling Performance in Response to Three Weeks of High-Intensity, Short Duration Overtraining, and a Two Week Taper. *The Sport Psychologist, 13*, 444-457.

Bortz, J. (1993). *Lehrbuch der Statistik für Sozialwissenschaftler* [Statistics for Social Scientists]. Berlin: Springer.

Boucsein, W. (1991). Arbeitspsychologische Beanspruchungsforschung heute - eine Herausforderung an die Psychologie [Work Psychological Stress Research - A Challenge for Psychology]. *Psychologische Rundschau, 42*, 129-144.

Bradburn, N.M. (1969). *The Structure of Physiological Well-Being*. Chicago: Aldine.

Budgett, R. (1998). Fatigue and Underperformance in Athletes: The Overtraining Syndrome. *British Journal of Sport and Medicine, 32*, 107-110.

Cohn, P. (1990). An Explanatory Study of Sources of Stress and Athlete Burnout in Youth Golf. *The Sport Psychologist, 4*, 95-106.

Dale, J., & Weinberg, R. (1989). The Relationship Between Coaches' Leadership Style and Burnout. *The Sport Psychologist, 3*, 1-13.

Debus, G., & Janke, W. (1978). Psychologische Aspekte der Psychopharmakotherapie [Psychological Aspects of Psychopharmaca Therapy]. In L.J. Pongratz (Ed.), *Handbuch der Psychologie* (Vol. 8, pp. 2161-2227). Göttingen: Hogrefe.

Diener, E., & Emmons, R. (1984). The Interpedendence of Positive and Negative Affect. *Journal of Personality and Social Psychology, 47*, 105-117.

Eberspächer, H. (1990). *Mentale Trainingsformen in der Praxis* [Applied Mental Training]. Oberhaching: Sportinform.

Eberspächer, H. (1995). *Mentales Training* [Mental Training]. München: Sportinform.

Eberspächer, H., & Kellmann, M. (1997). Trainingsformen zur Steigerung der Self-Efficacy im Sport [Drills and Exercises to Enhance Self-Efficacy in Sports]. In E. Christmann, J. Maxeiner, & D. Peper (Eds.), *Psychologische Aspekte beim Lernen, Trainieren und Realisieren sportlicher Bewegungshandlungen* (pp. 58-62). Köln: bps.

Eberspächer, H., Kellmann, M., & Hermann, H.-D. (1996). Kompetenzerwartung in sportlichen Beanspruchungssituationen [Self-Efficacy in Physically Stressful Situations]. In R. Daugs, K. Blischke, F. Marschall, & H. Müller (Eds.), *Kognition und Motorik* (pp. 153-159). Hamburg: Czwalina.

Erdmann, G., & Janke, W. (1981). *Mehrdimensionale Körperliche Symptomliste* [Multidimensional Physical Symptom List]. Unpublished Questionnaire. Berlin/Würzburg: Technical University of Berlin/University of Würzburg.

Feltz, D.L., Landers, D.M., & Reader, U. (1979). Enhancing Self-Efficacy in a High Avoidance Motor Task: A Comparison of Modeling Techniques. *Journal of Sport Psychology, 1*, 112-122.

Feltz, D.L., & Riessinger, C.A. (1990). Effects of in Vivo Emotive Imagery and Performance Feedback on Self-Efficacy and Muscular Endurance. *Journal of Sport & Exercise Psychology, 12*, 132-143.

Fender, L. (1989). Athlete Burnout: Potential for Research and Intervention Strategies. *The Sport Psychologist, 3*, 63-71.

Ferger, K. (1998a). Saisonbegleitende Diagnose der individuellen Belastungs-Erholungsbilanz mit der athletenspezifischen Variante des EBF [The Seasonal Diagnosis of the Individual Recovery-Stress State with the Sport-Specific Recovery-Stress Questionnaire]. In D. Teipel, R. Kemper, & D. Heinemann (Eds.), *Sportpsychologische Diagnostik, Prognostik und Intervention* (pp. 131-133). Köln: bps.

Ferger, K. (1998b). *Trainingseffekte im Fußball* [Training Effects in Soccer]. Hamburg: Feldhaus.

Fletcher, B. (1988). The Epidemiology of Occupational Stress. In C.L. Cooper & R. Payne (Eds.), *Causes, Coping, and Consequences of Stress at Work* (pp. 3-52). Chichester: Wiley.

Foster, C. (1998). Monitoring Training in Athletes with Reference to Overtraining Syndrome. *Medicine & Science in Sports and Exercise, 30*, 1164-1168.

Frese, M., & Zapf, D. (1994). Action as the Core of Work Psychology. A German Approach. In H.C. Triandis, M.D. Dunnette, & L.M. Hough (Eds.), *Handbook of Industrial and Organizational Psychology*, Vol. 4 (2nd. ed.) (pp. 271-340). Palo Alto, CA: Consulting Psychologists Press.

George, T.R., Feltz, D.L., & Chase, M.A. (1992). Effects of Model Similarity on Self-Efficacy and Muscular Endurance Performance: A Second Look. *Journal of Sport & Exercise Psychology, 14*, 237-248.

Hacker, W., & Richter, P. (1984). *Psychische Fehlbeanspruchung* [Psychological Over- and Understress]. Berlin: Springer.

Hagedorn, G. (1989). Die Auszeit im Sportspiel [Time-Out in Sport Games]. *Sportpsychologie, 3*, 26-28.

Hahn, E. (1978). Das Coachen von Fußballmannschaften in der Halbzeit [Coaching Soccer Teams During Half-Time]. *Leistungssport, 8*, 247-255.

Hahn, E. (1987). Erholungsrelevante Formen der Arbeitsorganisation bei rechnergestützer Bildschirmarbeit [Recovery-Related Forms of Work Organizations in Computer Settings]. *Sozialistische Arbeitswissenschaft, 31*, 338-349.

Hanin, Y.L. (1997). Emotions and Athletic Performance: Individual Zones of Optimal Functioning Model. In R. Seiler (Ed.), *European Yearbook of Sports Psychology* (Vol. 1, pp. 29-72). St. Augustin: Academia.

Hanin, Y.L. (2000). Individual Zones of Optimal Functioning (IZOF) Model: Emotion-Performance Relationships in Sport. In Y.L. Hanin (Ed.), *Emotions in Sport* (pp. 65-89). Champaign, IL: Human Kinetics.

Henschen, K. (1993). Athletic Staleness and Burnout: Diagnosis, Prevention, and Treatment. In J. Williams (Ed.), *Applied Sport Psychology* (pp. 328-337). Mountain View, CA: Mayfield Publishing Company.

Herzog, K., Voigt, H.F., & Westphal, G. (1985). *Volleyball-Training: Grundlagen und Arbeitshilfen* [Volleyball Training: Fundamentals and Applied Examples]. Schorndorf: Hofmann.

Hoffman, J.R., Epstein, S., Yarom, Y., Zigel, L., & Einbinder, M. (1999). Hormonal and Biochemical Changes in Elite Basketball Players During a 4-Week Training Camp. *Journal of Strength & Conditioning Research, 13*, 280-285.

Hogg, J.M. (2000). *Canadian Women's World Cup Soccer 1999: Mental Preparations. A report for Canadian Soccer Association*. Edmonton, Alberta: University of Alberta.

Hollmann, W. (1989). Ethische Gefahren im Hochleistungssport - Reflexionen aus sportmedizinischer Sicht [Ethical Dangers in Elite Sports - Reflexions from the Medical Perspective]. *Brennpunkte der Sportwissenschaft, 3*, 72-83.

Jagodzinski, W., Kühnel, S.M., & Schmidt, P. (1987). Is there a "Socratic Effect" in Nonexperimental Panel Studies? *Sociological Methods & Research, 15*, 259-302.

Janke, W. (1976). Psychophysische Grundlagen des Verhaltens [Psychophysic Fundamentals of Behavior]. In M. von Kerekjarto (Ed.), *Medizinische Psychologie* (pp. 1-101). Berlin: Springer.

Janke, W., & Wolffgramm, J. (1995). Biopsychologie von Streß und emotionalen Reaktionen: Ansätze interdisziplinärer Kooperation von Psychologie, Biologie und Medizin [Biopsychology of Stress and Emotional Reactions: Starting Points of an Interdisciplinary Cooperation of Psychology, Biology, and Medicine]. In G. Debus, G. Erdmann, & K.W. Kallus (Eds.), *Biospsychologie von Streß und emotionalen Reaktionen* (pp. 293-349). Göttingen: Hogrefe.

Jerusalem, M. (1990). *Persönliche Ressourcen, Vulnerabilität und Streßerleben* [Personal Resources, Vulnerability, and Stress Experience]. Göttingen: Hogrefe.

Jochum, M. (1994). *Untersuchungen des Beanspruchungszustandes und Spielleistung einer Basketball-Bundesligamannschaft* [Studies on the Recovery-Stress State and Performance of a First Division Basketball Team]. Unpublished thesis, Institut für Sport und Sportwissenschaft, Ruprecht-Karls-Universität, Heidelberg.

Kallus, K.W. (1992). *Beanspruchung und Ausgangszustand* [Stress and Initial State]. Weinheim: PVU.

Kallus, K.W. (1995). *Der Erholungs-Belastungs-Fragebogen* [The Recovery-Stress Questionnaire]. Frankfurt: Swets & Zeitlinger.

Kallus, K.W., Eberspächer, H., & Hermann, H.-D. (1992). Systematische, naive und gestörte Regeneration im Sport [Systematic, Naive and Disturbed Regeneration in Sports]. In L. Montada (Ed.), *Bericht über den 38. Kongreß der Deutschen Gesellschaft für Psychologie in Trier 1992* (Vol. 1: Kurzfassungen, pp. 436-437). Göttingen: Hogrefe.

Kallus, K.W., & Kellmann, M. (1995). The Recovery-Stress Questionnaire for Coaches. In R. Vanfraechem-Raway & Y. Vanden Auweele (Eds.), *Proceedings of the IXth European Congress on Sport Psychology in Brussels* (Part 1, pp. 26-33). Brussels: FEPSAC/Belgian Federation of Sport Psychology.

Kallus, K.W., & Kellmann, M. (2000). Burnout in Athletes and Coaches. In Y.L. Hanin (Ed.), *Emotions in Sport* (pp. 209-230). Champaign, IL: Human Kinetics.

Kallus, K.W., Kellmann, M., Eberspächer, H., & Hermann, H.-D. (1996). Beanspruchung, Erholung und Streßbewältigung von Trainern im Leistungssport [Stress, Recovery, and Coping with Stress of Coaches in Elite Sports]. *Psychologie und Sport, 3*, 114-126.

Kallus, K.W., & Krauth, J. (1995). Nichtparametrische Verfahren zum Nachweis emotionaler Reaktionen [Non-Parametric Methods for the Identification of Emotional Reactions]. In G. Debus, G. Erdmann, & K.W. Kallus (Eds.), *Biopsychologie von Streß und emotionalen Reaktionen* (pp. 23-43). Göttingen: Hogrefe.

Kanner, A.D., Coyne, J.C., Schaefer, C., & Lazarus, R. (1981). Comparison of Two Modes of Stress Management: Daily Hassles and Uplifts Versus Major Life Events. *Journal of Behavioral Medicine, 4*, 1-39.

Kellmann, M. (1991). *Die Abbildung des Beanspruchungszustandes durch den Erholungs-Belastungs-Fragebogen: Untersuchungen zur Leistungsprädiktion im Sport* [The Assessment of the Recovery-Stress State by the Recovery-Stress Questionnaire: Studies Dealing with Performance Prediction in Sports]. Unpublished Diploma thesis, Bayerische Julius-Maximilians-Universität, Würzburg.

Kellmann, M. (1997). *Die Wettkampfpause als integraler Bestandteil der Leistungsoptimierung im Sport: Eine empirische psychologische Analyse* [The Rest Period as an Integral Part of Optimizing Performance in Sports: An Empirical Psychological Analysis]. Hamburg: Kovac.

Kellmann, M. (1999). Die Beziehungen zwischen dem Erholungs-Belastungs-Fragebogen für Sportler und dem Profile of Mood States [The Relationships Between the Recovery-Stress Questionnaire for Athletes and the Profile of Mood States]. In D. Alfermann & O. Stoll (Eds.), *Motivation und Volition im Sport - Vom Planen zum Handeln* (pp. 208-212). Köln: bps.

Kellmann, M. (2000). Psychologische Methoden der Erholungs-Beanspruchungs-Diagnostik [Psychological Methods for the Assessment of Recovery and Stress]. *Deutsche Zeitschrift für Sportmedizin, 51,* 253-258.

Kellmann, M. (Ed.). (in press). *Optimal Recovery: Preventing Underperformance in Athletes.* Champaign, IL: Human Kinetics.

Kellmann, M., & Altenburg, D. (2000). Betreuung der Junioren-Nationalmannschaft des Deutschen Ruderverbandes [Consultation of the German Junior National Rowing Team]. In H. Allmer, W. Hartmann, & D. Kayser (Eds.), *Sportpsychologie in Bewegung - Forschung für die Praxis* (pp. 67-80). Köln: Sport und Buch Strauss.

Kellmann, M., Altenburg, D., Lormes, W., & Steinacker, J.M. (2001). Assessing Stress and Recovery during Preparation for the World Championships in Rowing. *The Sport Psychologist, 15,* 151-167.

Kellmann, M., Fritzenberg, M., & Beckmann, J. (2000). Erfassung von Belastung und Erholung im Behindertensport [Assessment of Stress and Recovery in Sport with Athletes with a Physical Handicap]. *Psychologie und Sport, 7,* 141-152.

Kellmann, M., Gould, D., Smith, D.J., Botterill, C., Blakeley, A., McCann, S.C., & Wrisberg, C.A. (1999). Overtraining in Sport (Symposium). *Abstracts of the 14th Conference of the Association for the Advancement of Applied Sport Psychology (AAASP) from the 22 - 26 September 1999 in Banff, Alberta. Abstracts (pp. 12-13).* Banff: AAASP.

Kellmann, M., & Günther, K.-D. (1999). Die Diagnose der Erholungs-Beanspruchungs-Bilanz während des WM-Trainingslagers des DRV [The Recovery-Stress-Balance Diagnosis During Competition Preparation]. In W. Fritsch (Ed.), *Rudern - informieren, reflektieren, innovieren* (pp. 287-293). Wiebelsheim: Limpert.

Kellmann, M., & Günther, K.-D. (2000). Changes in Stress and Recovery in Elite Rowers During Preparation for the Olympic Games. *Medicine & Science in Sports and Exercise, 32,* 676-683.

Kellmann, M., Johnson, M.S., & Wrisberg, C.A. (1998). Auswirkungen der Erholungs-Beanspruchungs-Bilanz auf die Wettkampfleistung von amerikanischen Schwimmerinnen [The Effects That the Recovery-Stress State Has on the Performance of American Female Swimmers]. In D. Teipel, R. Kemper, & D. Heinemann (Eds.), *Sportpsychologische Diagnostik, Prognostik und Intervention* (pp. 123-126). Köln: bps.

Kellmann, M., & Kallus, K.W. (1993). The Recovery-Stress Questionnaire: A Potential Tool to Predict Performance in Sports. In J.R. Nitsch & R. Seiler (Eds.), *Movement and Sport: Psychological Foundations and Effects* (Vol. 1, pp. 242-247). Sankt Augustin: Academia.

Kellmann, M., & Kallus, K.W. (1994). Interrelation Between Stress and Coaches' Behavior During Rest Periods. *Perceptual and Motor Skills, 79,* 207-210.

Kellmann, M., & Kallus, K.W. (1995). The Rest-Period-Questionnaire for Coaches: Assessing the Behavior of Coaches During Rest Periods. In R. Vanfraechem-Raway & Y. Vanden Auweele (Eds.), *Proceedings of the IXth European Congress on Sport Psychology* (Part 1, pp. 43-50). Brussels: FEPSAC / Belgian Federation of Sport Psychology.

Kellmann, M., & Kallus, K.W. (1999). Mood, Recovery-Stress State, and Regeneration. In M. Lehmann, C. Foster, U. Gastmann, H. Keizer, & J.M. Steinacker (Eds.), *Overload, Fatigue, Performance Incompetence, and Regeneration in Sport* (pp. 101-117). New York: Plenum.

Kellmann, M., & Kallus, K.W. (2000). *Der Erholungs-Belastungs-Fragebogen für Sportler; Handanweisung* [The Recovery-Stress Questionnaire for Athletes; Manual]. Frankfurt: Swets Test Services.

Kellmann, M., Kallus, K.W., Günther, K.-D., Lormes, W., & Steinacker, J.M. (1997). Psychologische Betreuung der Junioren-Nationalmannschaft des Deutschen Ruderverbandes [Psychological Consultation of the German Junior National Rowing Team]. *Psychologie und Sport, 4,* 123-134.

Kellmann, M., Kallus, K.W., & Kurz, H. (1996). Performance Prediction by the Recovery-Stress Questionnaire. *Journal of Applied Sport Psychology, 8,* Supplement, S22.

Kellmann, M., Kallus, K.W., Steinacker, J., & Lormes, W. (1997). Monitoring Stress and Recovery During the Training Camp for the Junior World Championships in Rowing. *Journal of Applied Sport Psychology, 8,* Supplement, S114.

Kenttä, G., & Hassmén, P. (1998). Overtraining and Recovery. *Sports Medicine, 26,* 1-16.

Krauth, J. (1995). *Testkonstruktion und Testtheorie* [Development and Theory of Tests]. Weinheim: PVU.

Kuhl, J., & Fuhrmann, A. (1998). Decomposing Self-Regulation and Self-Control: The Volitional Components Inventory. In J. Heckhausen & C. Dweck (Eds.), *Life Span Perspectives on Motivation and Control* (pp. 15-49). Cambridge: Cambridge University Press.

Kuipers, H. (1998). Training and Overtraining: An Introduction. *Medicine & Science in Sports and Exercise, 30,* 1137-1139.

Kuipers, H., & Keizer, H.A. (1988). Overtraining in Elite Athletes: Review and Directions for the Future. *Sports Medicine, 6*, 79-92.

Kurz, H. (1995). *Beanspruchungsoptimierung bei Schwimmern* [Optimizing Stress of Swimmers]. Unpublished thesis, Sporthochschule, Köln.

Laux, L. (1983). Psychologische Streßkonzeptionen [Psychological Stress Concepts]. In H. Thomae (Ed.), *Enzyklopädie der Psychologie* (Bd. IV/1, pp. 453-535). Göttingen: Hogrefe.

Lazarus, R.S. (1991). *Emotion and Adaptation.* New York: Oxford University Press.

Lazarus, R.S., & Launier, R. (1978). Stress-Related Transactions Between Person and Environment. In R. Plutchik & M. Lewis (Eds.), *Perspectives in International Psychology* (pp. 287-327). New York: Plenum.

Lehmann, M.J., Foster, C., Dickhut, H.-H., & Gastmann, U. (1998). Autonomic Imbalance Hypothesis and Overtraining Syndrome. *Medicine & Science in Sports and Exercise, 30*, 1140-1145.

Lehmann, M.J., Foster, C., Gastmann, U., Keizer, H.A., & Steinacker, J.M. (1999). Definition, Types, Symptoms, Findings, Underlying Mechanisms, and Frequency of Overtraining and Overtraining Syndrome. In M.J. Lehmann, C. Foster, U. Gastmann, H. Keizer, & J.M. Steinacker (Eds.), *Overload, Fatigue, Performance Incompetence, and Regeneration in Sport* (pp. 1-6). New York: Plenum.

Lehmann, M., Foster, C., & Keul, J. (1993). Overtraining in Endurance Athletes: A Brief Review. *Medicine & Science in Sports and Exercise, 25*, 854-861.

Lehmann, M.J., Foster, C., Netzer, N., Lormes, W., Steinacker, J.M., Lui, Y., Opitz-Gress, A., & Gastmann, U. (1998). Physiological Responses to Short- and Long-Term Overtraining in Endurance Athletes. In R.B. Kreider, A.C. Fry, & M.L. O'Toole (Eds.), *Overtraining in Sport* (pp. 19-46). Champaign, IL: Human Kinetics.

Lehmann, M.J., Lormes, W., Opitz-Gress, A., Steinacker, J.M., Netzer, N., Foster, C., & Gastmann, U. (1997). Training and Overtraining: An Overview and Experimental Results in Endurance Sports. *The Journal of Sports Medicine and Physical Fitness, 37*, 7-17.

Lienert, G.A. (1969). *Testaufbau und Testanalyse* [Development and Analysis of Tests]. Weinheim: Beltz.

Lienert, G.A. (1973). *Verteilungsfreie Methoden in der Biostatistik* [Distribution Free Methods in Bio-Statistics]. Meisenheim: Anton Hain.

Lienert, G.A., & Raatz, U. (1994). *Testaufbau und Testanalyse* [Development and Analysis of Tests]. Weinheim: Beltz, PVU.

Löhr, G., & Preiser, S. (1974). Regression und Recreation - Ein Beitrag zum Problem Streß und Erholung [Regression and Recreation - A Paper Dealing with Stress and Recovery]. *Zeitschrift für experimentelle und angewandte Psychologie, 21*, 575-591.

Martin, D.T., Andersen, M.B., & Gates, W. (2000). Using Profile of Mood States (POMS) to Monitor High-Intensity Training in Cyclists: Group versus Case Studies. *The Sport Psychologist, 14*, 138-156.

Maslach, C., & Jackson, S.E. (1986). *Maslach Burnout Inventory.* Palo Alto, CA: Consulting Psychologists Press.

McAuley, E. (1985). Modeling and Self-Efficacy: A Test of Bandura's Model. *Journal of Sport Psychology, 7*, 283-295.

McNair, D., Lorr, M., & Droppleman, L.F. (1971). *Profile of Mood States Manual.* San Diego: Educational and Industrial Testing Service.

McNair, D., Lorr, M., & Droppleman, L.F. (1992). *Profile of Mood States Manual.* San Diego: Educational and Industrial Testing Service.

Moosbrugger, H. (1982). Dimensionalitätsuntersuchungen von FPI-Skalen mit dem Klassisch-Latent-Additiven Testmodell (KLA-Modell) [Studies of Dimensionality by FPI-Scales With the Classical-Latent-Additive Test Model]. *Zeitschrift für Differentielle und Diagnostische Psychologie, 3*, 241-264.

Morgan, W.P. (1985). Selected Psychological Factors Limiting Performance: A Mental Health Model. In D.H. Clarke & H.M. Eckert (Eds.), *Limits of Human Performance* (pp. 70-80). Champaign, IL: Human Kinetics.

Morgan, W.P., Brown, D.R., Raglin, J.S., O'Conner, P.J., & Ellickson, K.A. (1987). Psychological Monitoring of Overtraining and Staleness. *British Journal of Sport Medicine, 21*, 107-114.

Morgan, W.P., & Costill, D.L. (1996). Selected Psychological Characteristics and Health Behaviors of Aging Marathon Runners: A Longitudinal Study. *International Journal of Sport Medicine, 17*, 305-312.

Morgan, W.P., Costill, D.L., Flynn, M.G., Raglin, J.S., & O'Conner, P. (1988). Mood Disturbance Following Increased Training in Swimmers. *Medicine & Science in Sports and Exercise, 20*, 408-414.

Odom, S., & Perrin, T. (1985). Coach and Athlete Burnout. In L. Bunker, R. Rotella, & A. Reilly (Eds.), *Sport Psychology: Psychological Considerations in Maximizing Sport Performance* (pp. 213-222). Ann Arbor, MI: McDaught and Quinn Inc.

Pines, A. (1993). Burnout. In L. Goldberger & S. Breznitz (Eds.), *Handbook of Stress* (pp. 386-402). New York: The Free Press.

Raglin, J.S. (1993). Overtraining and Staleness: Psychometric Monitoring of Endurance Athletes. In R.B. Singer, M. Murphey, & L.K. Tennant (Eds.), *Handbook of Research on Sport Psychology* (pp. 840-850). New York: Macmillan.

Renzland, J., & Eberspächer, H. (1988). *Regeneration im Sport* [Regeneration in Sports]. Köln: bps.

Rieder, H., Riffelt, D., & Vierneisel, S. (1988). Regeneration nach sportlicher Belastung [Regeneration After Physical Stress]. *Leistungssport, 18*, 8-15.

Robinson, T., & Carron, A. (1982). Personal and Situational Factors Associated With Dropping Out Versus Maintaining Participation in Competitive Sport. *Journal of Sport Psychology, 4*, 364-378.

Rohmert, W., & Rutenfranz, J. (1975). *Arbeitswissenschaftliche Beurteilung der Belastung und Beanspruchung an unterschiedlichen industriellen Arbeitsplätzen* [Scientific Rating on Stress in Different Industrial Workplaces]. Bonn: Bundesminister für Arbeit und Sozialordnung.

Rüger, U., Blomert, A.F., & Förster, W. (1990). *Coping. Theoretische Konzepte, Forschungsansätze, Meßinstrumente zur Krankheitsbewältigung* [Coping. Theoretical Concepts, Research Designs, and Instruments for Dealing With Illness]. Göttingen: Verlag für Medizinische Psychologie im Verlag Vandenhoeck & Ruprecht.

Savis, J.C. (1994). Sleep and Athletic Performance: Overview and Implications for Sport Psychology. *The Sport Psychologist, 8*, 111-125.

Schönpflug, W. (1983). Coping Efficiency and Situational Demands. In R. Hockey (Ed.), *Stress and Fatigue in Human Performance* (pp. 299-326). Chichester: Wiley.

Schönpflug, W. (1987). Beanspruchung und Belastung bei der Arbeit - Konzepte und Theorien. Arbeitspsychologie [Strain and Stress During Work - Concepts and Theories]. In U. Kleinbeck & J. Rutenfranz (Eds.), *Enzyklopädie der Psychologie* (Part III/1, pp. 131-184). Göttingen: Hogrefe.

Smith, R.E. (1986). Toward a Cognitive-Affective Model of Athletic Burnout. *Journal of Sport Psychology, 8*, 36-50.

Smith, R.E. (1989). Athletic Stress and Burnout: Conceptual Models and Intervention Strategies. In D. Hackfort & C.D. Spielberger (Eds.), *Anxiety in Sports: An International Perspective* (pp. 183-202). New York: Hemisphere Publishing Corporation.

Spielberger, C.D., Gorsuch, R.L., & Lushene, R.E. (1970). *Manual for the State-Trait Anxiety Inventory (STAI)*. Palo Alto, CA: Consulting Psychologists Press.

Spink, K.S. (1990). Group Cohesion and Collective Efficacy of Volleyball Teams. *Journal of Sport & Exercise Psychology, 12*, 301-311.

Sprung, L., & Sprung, H. (1987). *Grundlagen der Methodologie und Methodik der Psychologie* [Fundamentals of the Methods in Psychology]. Berlin: Deutscher Verlag der Wissenschaften.

Steinacker, J.M. (1993). Physiological Aspects of Training in Rowing. *International Journal of Sports Medicine, 14*, S3-S10.

Steinacker, J.M., Kellmann, M., Böhm, B.O., Liu, Y., Opitz-Gress, A., Kallus, K.W., Lehmann, M., Altenburg, D., &

Lormes, W. (1999). Clinical Findings and Parameters of Stress and Regeneration in Rowers Before World Championships. In M. Lehmann, C. Foster, U. Gastmann, H. Keizer, & J.M. Steinacker (Eds.), *Overload, Fatigue, Performance Incompetence, and Regeneration in Sport* (pp. 71-80). New York: Plenum.

Steinacker, J.M., Laske, R., Hetzel, W.D., Lormes, W., Liu, Y., & Strauch, M. (1993). Metabolic and Hormonal Reactions During Training in Junior Oarsmen. *International Journal of Sports Medicine, 14*, S24-S28.

Steinacker, J.M., Lormes, W., Kellmann, M., Liu, Y., Reißnecker, S., Opitz-Gress, A., Baller, B., Günther, K., Petersen, K.G., Kallus, K.W., Lehmann, M., & Altenburg, D. (2000). Training of Junior Rowers Before World Championships. Effects on Performance, Mood State and Selected Hormonal and Metabolic Responses. *Journal of Sports Medicine and Physical Fitness, 40*, 327-335.

Steinacker, J.M., Lormes, W., Lehmann, M., & Altenburg, D. (1998). Training of Rowers Before World Championships. *Medicine & Science in Sports and Exercise, 30*, 1158-1163.

Stone, A.A., & Neale, M. (1984). Effects of Severe Daily Events on Mood. *Journal of Personality and Social Psychology, 46*, 137-144.

Vroom, V.H. (1964). *Work and Motivation*. New York: Wiley.

Weineck, J. (1994). *Optimales Training* [Optimal Training]. Erlangen: perimed.

Weyer, G., & Hodapp, V. (1975). Entwicklung von Fragebogenskalen zur Erfassung der subjektiven Belastung [Development of a Questionnaire for the Assessment of Subjective Stress]. *Archiv für Psychologie, 127*, 161-188.

Wieland-Eckelmann, R., & Baggen, R. (1994). Beanspruchung und Erholung im Arbeits-Erholungs-Zyklus [Stress and Recovery in the Work-Recovery Cycle]. In R. Wieland-Eckelmann, H. Allmer, K.W. Kallus, & J. Otto (Eds.), *Erholungsforschung* (pp. 102-154). Weinheim: PVU.

Wilhelm, A., & Janssen, J.P. (1989). Beanspruchung und Belastung im Triathlon [Strain and Stress in Triathlon]. *Sportpsychologie, 3*, 18-22.

Wittig, A.F., Duncan, S.L., & Schnurr, K.T. (1987). The Relationship of Gender, Gender-Role Endorsement, and Perceived Physical Self-Efficacy to Sport Competition Anxiety. *Journal of Sport Behavior, 10*, 192-199.

About the Authors

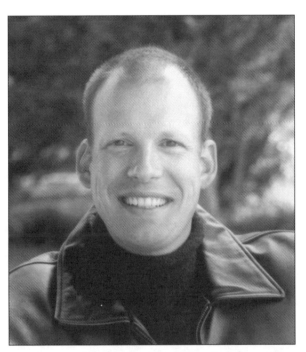

Michael Kellmann, PhD, is a Hochschulassistent (assistant professor) of sport psychology at the University of Potsdam Institute of Sport Science in Potsdam, Germany.

Dr. Kellmann is a member of the Association for the Advancement of Applied Sport Psychology (AAASP), the German Association of Sport Psychology, and Psychology in High Performance Sports. He serves on the editorial board for *The Sport Psychologist* and his works have appeared in more than 50 publications. He has consulted with and conducted research for the National Sport Center in Calgary, Canada, the Canadian national speed skating team, and the German Junior national rowing team.

Dr. Kellmann lives in Potsdam, Germany, and enjoys running and playing soccer.

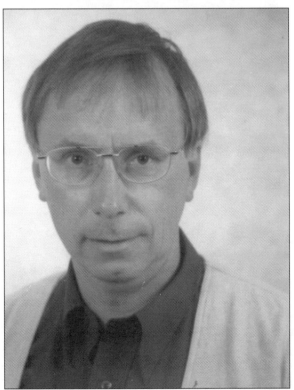

K. Wolfgang Kallus, PhD, is a full professor of work, organizational, and environmental psychology at the University of Graz in Graz, Austria, and is a member of the directorate of the Institute for Evaluation Research in Germany.

Dr. Kallus is on the editorial board of *Neuropsychobiology.* He is a member of the International Biometric Society and the Collegium Neuropsychopharmacology. His work focuses on stress, coping, and regeneration in applications as diverse as sport, work, surgery, and aviation.

Dr. Kallus lives in Graz, Austria. He enjoys spending time with his family, canoeing, and skiing.

Appendix A

<table>
<tr><td colspan="2">Table A1</td><td colspan="7">Overview of the Items of the Recovery-Stress Questionnaire for Athletes in the RESTQ Basic Modules (RESTQ-24A, RESTQ-24B, and RESTQ-48), the Various Developmental Versions (RESTQ-86, RESTQ-85, RESTQ-80), the Regular Version (RESTQ-76), and the Short Version (RESTQ-52)</td></tr>
</table>

Scale 1: General Stress	24A	24B	48	86	85	80	76	52
. . . I felt down	14	–	22	22	22	22	22	14
. . . I felt depressed	–	11	24	24	24	24	24	–
. . . I was fed up with everything	16	–	30	30	30	30	30	16
. . . everything was too much for me	–	21	45	45	45	45	45	–

Scale 2: Emotional Stress	24A	24B	48	86	85	80	76	52
. . . I was in a bad mood	3	–	8	8	8	8	8	3
. . . everything bothered me	–	5	5	5	5	5	5	–
. . . I felt anxious or inhibited	–	24	28	28	28	28	28	–
. . . I was annoyed	20	–	37	37	37	37	37	20

Scale 3: Social Stress	24A	24B	48	86	85	80	76	52
. . . I was annoyed by others	13	–	21	21	21	21	21	13
. . . other people got on my nerves	–	13	26	26	26	26	26	–
. . . I was upset	22	–	39	39	39	39	39	22
. . . I was angry with someone	–	24	48	48	48	48	48	–

Scale 4: Conflicts/Pressure	24A	24B	48	86	85	80	76	52
. . . I was worried about unresolved problems	7	–	12	12	12	12	12	7
. . . I couldn't switch my mind off	–	8	18	18	18	18	18	–
. . . I felt I had to perform well in front of others	–	17	32	32	32	32	32	–
. . . I felt under pressure	25	–	44	44	44	44	44	25

Scale 5: Fatigue	24A	24B	48	86	85	80	76	52
. . . I did not get enough sleep	–	2	2	2	2	2	2	–
. . . I was tired from work	–	12	25	25	25	25	25	–
. . . I was dead tired after work	10	–	16	16	16	16	16	10
. . . I was overtired	18	–	35	35	35	35	35	18

(continued)

Scale 6: Lack of Energy	24A	24B	48	86	85	80	76	52
. . . I was unable to concentrate well	–	4	4	4	4	4	4	–
. . . I had difficulties in concentrating	6	–	11	11	11	11	11	6
. . . I was lethargic	–	16	31	31	31	31	31	–
. . . I put off making decisions	23	–	40	40	40	40	40	23

Scale 7: Physical Complaints	24A	24B	48	86	85	80	76	52
. . . I felt physically bad	–	6	7	7	7	7	7	–
. . . I had a headache	9	–	15	15	15	15	15	9
. . . I felt uncomfortable	12	–	20	20	20	20	20	12
. . . I felt physically exhausted	–	19	42	42	42	42	42	–

Scale 8: Success	24A	24B	48	86	85	80	76	52
. . . I finished important tasks	–	3	3	3	3	3	3	–
. . . I was successful in what I did	11	–	17	17	17	17	17	11
. . . I made important decisions	24	–	41	41	41	41	41	24
. . . I had some good ideas	–	25	49	49	49	49	49	–

Scale 9: Social Recovery	24A	24B	48	86	85	80	76	52
. . . I laughed	2	–	6	6	6	6	6	2
. . . I had fun	–	18	33	33	33	33	33	–
. . . I had a good time with my friends	8	–	14	14	14	14	14	8
. . . I visited some close friends	–	10	23	23	23	23	23	–

Scale 10: Physical Recovery	24A	24B	48	86	85	80	76	52
. . . I felt physically fit	–	15	29	29	29	29	29	–
. . . I felt at ease	–	7	13	13	13	13	13	–
. . . I felt physically relaxed	4	–	9	9	9	9	9	4
. . . I felt as if I could get everything done	21	–	38	38	38	38	38	21

Scale 11: General Well-Being	24A	24B	48	86	85	80	76	52
. . . I was in good spirits	5	–	10	10	10	10	10	5
. . . I was in a good mood	17	–	34	34	34	34	34	17
. . . I felt happy	–	20	43	43	43	43	43	–
. . . I felt content	–	23	47	47	47	47	47	–

Scale 12: Sleep Quality	24A	24B	48	86	85	80	76	52
. . . my sleep was interrupted easily	–	22	46	46	46	46	46	–
. . . I slept restlessly	19	–	36	36	36	36	36	19
. . . I had a satisfying sleep	15	–	27	27	27	27	27	15
. . . I fell asleep satisfied and relaxed	–	9	19	19	19	19	19	–

Scale 13: Disturbed Breaks	24A	24B	48	86	85	80	76	52
. . . I used my breaks during practice consciously	–	–	–	67	–	–	–	–
. . . I felt disturbed in my breaks during practice	–	–	–	82	–	–	–	–
. . . at the end of the breaks, I prepared myself well for the next stage of performance	–	–	–	–	76	–	–	–
. . . I had the impression there were too few breaks	–	–	–	–	50	58	58	34
. . . my coach demanded too much of me during the breaks	–	–	–	–	57	–	–	–
. . . too much was demanded of me during the breaks	–	–	–	–	–	66	66	42
. . . the breaks were not at the right times	–	–	–	–	67	72	72	48
. . . the coach did not leave me alone during the breaks	–	–	–	–	80	–	–	–
. . . I could not get rest during the breaks	–	–	–	–	–	51	51	27

Scale 14: Emotional Exhaustion	24A	24B	48	86	85	80	76	52
. . . I felt that I had to practice too much	–	–	–	57	–	–	–	–
. . . I felt burned out by my sport	–	–	–	68	65	54	54	30
. . . I felt exhausted after practice	–	–	–	70	–	–	–	–
. . . I felt that I wanted to quit my sport	–	–	–	75	73	68	68	44
. . . I felt frustrated by my sport	–	–	–	81	75	76	76	52
. . . I felt emotionally drained from performance	–	–	–	86	78	63	63	39

Scale 15: Injury	24A	24B	48	86	85	80	76	52
. . . I had muscle pain after performance	–	–	–	50	51	64	64	40
. . . I felt vulnerable to injuries	–	–	–	54	54	73	73	49
. . . I didn't warm up properly	–	–	–	59	–	–	–	–
. . . I got injured	–	–	–	65	–	–	–	–

(continued)

	24A	24B	48	86	85	80	76	52
. . . parts of my body were aching	–	–	–	72	70	50	50	26
. . . practice drained my body	–	–	–	79	74	–	–	–
. . . my muscles felt stiff or tense during performance	–	–	–	–	62	57	57	33
. . . I felt exhausted after performance	–	–	–	–	68	–	–	–

Scale 16: Being in Shape	**24A**	**24B**	**48**	**86**	**85**	**80**	**76**	**52**
. . . I felt very energetic	–	–	–	–	55	69	69	45
. . . I felt physically fit	–	–	–	61	–	–	–	–
. . . I recovered well physically	–	–	–	66	63	53	53	29
. . . my body was relaxed	–	–	–	74	–	–	–	–
. . . my body felt strong	–	–	–	–	72	75	75	51
. . . I felt unstoppable	–	–	–	77	–	–	–	–
. . . I had a flowing experience in practice	–	–	–	80	–	–	–	–
. . . I felt that my body was working without my mind	–	–	–	85	–	–	–	–
. . . I was in a good condition physically	–	–	–	–	58	61	61	37

Scale 17: Personal Accomplishment	**24A**	**24B**	**48**	**86**	**85**	**80**	**76**	**52**
. . . I dealt with emotional problems in my sport very calmly	–	–	–	52	52	77	77	53
. . . I felt very energetic	–	–	–	56	–	–	–	–
. . . I easily understood how my teammates felt about things	–	–	–	62	59	70	70	46
. . . I accomplished many worthwhile things in my sport	–	–	–	69	66	55	55	31
. . . I delt very effectively with my teammates' problems	–	–	–	73	71	60	60	36
. . . I felt that all I wanted to do is my sport	–	–	–	84	77	–	–	–

Scale 18: Self-Efficacy	**24A**	**24B**	**48**	**86**	**85**	**80**	**76**	**52**
. . . I was convinced that I performed well	–	–	–	–	81	65	65	41
. . . I was convinced I did the right thing	–	–	–	–	82	–	–	–
. . . I was convinced that I was ready for any problem that should come up	–	–	–	–	83	–	–	–
. . . I was convinced I could achieve my set goals during performance	–	–	–	–	84	–	–	–

. . . I was convinced that I had trained well	–	–	–	–	85	71	71	47
. . . I was convinced that I could achieve my performance at any time	–	–	–	–	86	–	–	–
. . . I was convinced that I could achieve my set goals during performance	–	–	–	–	–	52	52	28
. . . I was convinced that I could achieve my performance at any time	–	–	–	–	–	59	59	35

Scale 19: Self-Regulation	**24A**	**24B**	**48**	**86**	**85**	**80**	**76**	**52**
. . . I was talking positively to myself during practice	–	–	–	58	–	–	–	–
. . . I pushed myself during performance	–	–	–	53	53	62	62	38
. . . I was convinced that I was doing well in practice	–	–	–	63	–	–	–	–
. . . I was convinced that I had trained well	–	–	–	–	60	–	–	–
. . . I believed in what I did during practice	–	–	–	78	–	–	–	–
. . . I could concentrate when I wanted to	–	–	–	55	–	–	–	–
. . . I could focus my attention whenever I wanted to	–	–	–	87	79	–	–	–
. . . I psyched myself up before performance	–	–	–	71	69	67	67	43
. . . I was able to monitor my body	–	–	–	83	–	–	–	–
. . . I prepared myself mentally for performance	–	–	–	64	61	56	56	32
. . . mental training was a part of my day	–	–	–	76	–	–	–	–
. . . I talked with my coach how I performed lately	–	–	–	51	–	–	–	–
. . . I was setting goals for myself	–	–	–	60	–	–	–	–
. . . I set definite goals for myself during performance	–	–	–	–	56	74	74	50

Table A2 Mean (M), Standard Deviation (SD), and Correted Item Total Correlation (r$_{(i;t-i)}$) of the RESTQ-76 Sport for the Canadian C2 (bold; n = 128) and the German R1-3 (n = 128) Samples

Scale 1: General Stress

No.	Item	M	SD	r$_{(i;t-i)}$
22)	. . . I felt down	1.75 **1.65**	1.13 **1.41**	.50 **.83**
24)	. . . I felt depressed	1.36 **1.29**	1.05 **1.61**	.52 **.78**
30)	. . . I was fed up with everything	1.42 **1.30**	1.25 **1.39**	.60 **.80**
45)	. . . everything was too much for me	1.36 **1.38**	1.16 **1.44**	.64 **.76**

Scale 2: Emotional Stress

No.	Item	M	SD	r$_{(i;t-i)}$
5)	. . . everything bothered me	1.87 **1.57**	1.02 **1.32**	.50 **.76**
8)	. . . I was in a bad mood	1.71 **1.65**	.88 **1.28**	.60 **.72**
28)	. . . I felt anxious or inhibited	.76 **1.99**	1.02 **1.48**	.29 **.52**
37)	. . . I was annoyed	2.07 **1.67**	1.03 **1.26**	.63 **.72**

Scale 3: Social Stress

No.	Item	M	SD	r$_{(i;t-i)}$
21)	. . . I was annoyed by others	2.30 **1.98**	1.06 **1.55**	.71 **.81**
26)	. . . other people got on my nerves	2.24 **1.72**	1.13 **1.36**	.76 **.84**
39)	. . . I was upset	1.71 **1.54**	1.06 **1.40**	.56 **.70**
48)	. . . I was angry with someone	1.58 **1.41**	1.07 **1.51**	.75 **.78**

Scale 4: Conflicts/Pressure

No.	Item	M	SD	$r_{(i;t-i)}$
12)	. . . I was worried about unresolved problems	1.40 **2.77**	1.25 **1.61**	.43 **.65**
18)	. . . I couldn't switch my mind off	2.71 **2.27**	1.45 **1.65**	.46 **.55**
32)	. . . I felt I had to perform well in front of others	1.95 **2.64**	1.48 **1.71**	.49 **.64**
44)	. . . I felt under pressure	2.69 **2.28**	1.26 **1.69**	.48 **.66**

Scale 5: Fatigue

No.	Item	M	SD	$r_{(i;t-i)}$
2)	. . . I did not get enough sleep	1.89 **2.38**	1.07 **1.48**	.53 **.48**
16)	. . . I was tired from work	3.28 **2.20**	1.24 **1.69**	.61 **.64**
25)	. . . I was dead tired after work	3.11 **1.71**	1.37 **1.66**	.65 **.79**
35)	. . . I was overtired	1.87 **2.05**	1.20 **1.53**	.57 **.68**

Scale 6: Lack of Energy

No.	Item	M	SD	$r_{(i;t-i)}$
4)	. . . I was unable to concentrate well	1.73 **2.07**	.73 **1.23**	.56 **.72**
11)	. . . I had difficulties in concentrating	1.66 **2.01**	.76 **1.24**	.58 **.75**
31)	. . . I was lethargic	1.36 **2.06**	.92 **1.69**	.59 **.59**
40)	. . . I put off making decisions	1.01 **2.12**	.92 **1.55**	.34 **.62**

(continued)

Scale 7: Physical Complaints

No.	Item	M	SD	$r_{(i;t-i)}$
7)	. . . I felt physically bad	1.91	1.15	.59
		2.30	**1.43**	**.63**
15)	. . . I had a headache	.62	1.03	.32
		1.25	**1.62**	**.46**
20)	. . . I felt uncomfortable	1.85	1.14	.61
		1.82	**1.45**	**.57**
42)	. . . I felt physically exhausted	2.53	1.13	.50
		2.08	**1.54**	**.58**

Scale 8: Success

No.	Item	M	SD	$r_{(i;t-i)}$
3)	. . . I finished important tasks	2.23	1.33	.38
		3.52	**1.54**	**.61**
17)	. . . I was successful in what I did	2.71	1.03	.51
		3.48	**1.32**	**.61**
41)	. . . I made important decisions	1.71	1.18	.55
		2.38	**1.40**	**.48**
49)	. . . I had some good ideas	2.27	.94	.41
		3.08	**1.32**	**.65**

Scale 9: Social Recovery

No.	Item	M	SD	$r_{(i;t-i)}$
6)	. . . I laughed	4.13	.89	.59
		3.89	**1.51**	**.67**
14)	. . . I had a good time with my friends	3.77	1.03	.72
		3.63	**1.39**	**.83**
23)	. . . I visited some close friends	3.87	1.44	.53
		2.66	**1.78**	**.60**
33)	. . . I had fun	4.01	.93	.74
		3.84	**1.42**	**.76**

Scale 10: Physical Recovery

No.	Item	M	SD	$r_{(i;t-i)}$
9)	. . . I felt physically relaxed	2.52 **2.99**	1.08 **1.43**	.71 **.68**
13)	. . . I felt at ease	2.91 **3.02**	1.09 **1.41**	.65 **.72**
29)	. . . I felt physically fit	3.26 **3.09**	1.09 **1.55**	.77 **.64**
38)	. . . I felt as if I could get everything done	3.40 **2.65**	1.10 **1.46**	.64 **.60**

Scale 11: General Well-Being

No.	Item	M	SD	$r_{(i;t-i)}$
10)	. . . I was in good spirits	3.51 **3.76**	1.01 **1.37**	.57 **.84**
34)	. . . I was in a good mood	3.95 **3.67**	.91 **1.30**	.72 **.88**
43)	. . . I felt happy	3.28 **3.71**	1.13 **1.45**	.71 **.88**
47)	. . . I felt content	3.27 **3.44**	1.09 **1.46**	.70 **.76**

Scale 12: Sleep Quality

No.	Item	M	SD	$r_{(i;t-i)}$
19)	. . . I fell asleep satisfied and relaxed	3.32 **3.07**	1.41 **1.52**	.65 **.61**
27)	. . . I had a satisfying sleep	3.74 **3.03**	1.27 **1.55**	.68 **.76**
36)	. . . I slept restlessly	4.43 **4.17**	1.35 **1.76**	.72 **.76**
46)	. . . my sleep was interrupted easily	5.13 **4.28**	1.18 **1.74**	.58 **.70**

Scale 13: Disturbed Breaks

No.	Item	M	SD	$r_{(i;t-i)}$
51)	. . . I could not get rest during the breaks	1.10 **2.07**	1.10 **1.54**	.59 **.49**
58)	. . . I had the impression there were too few breaks	1.59 **1.55**	1.07 **1.67**	.60 **.75**
66)	. . . too much was demanded of me during the breaks	.88 **1.69**	1.01 **1.63**	.73 **.71**
72)	. . . the breaks were not at the right times	1.05 **1.38**	.98 **1.44**	.52 **.73**

Scale 14: Burnout/Emotional Exhaustion

No.	Item	M	SD	$r_{(i;t-i)}$
54)	. . . I felt burned out by my sport	2.40 **1.35**	1.22 **1.55**	.49 **.77**
63)	. . . I felt emotionally drained from performance	1.93 **1.94**	1.15 **1.61**	.51 **.69**
68)	. . . I felt that I wanted to quit my sport	.50 **.77**	1.02 **1.50**	.50 **.75**
76)	. . . I felt frustrated by my sport	1.22 **1.78**	1.04 **1.83**	.48 **.66**

Scale 15: Fitness/Injury

No.	Item	M	SD	$r_{(i;t-i)}$
50)	. . . parts of my body were aching	2.36 **2.77**	1.36 **1.76**	.63 **.69**
57)	. . . my muscles felt stiff or tense during performance	2.00 **2.57**	1.45 **1.65**	.64 **.63**
64)	. . . I had muscle pain after performance	2.11 **2.56**	1.34 **1.75**	.63 **.64**
73)	. . . I felt vulnerable to injuries	1.17 **2.01**	1.09 **1.97**	.48 **.59**

Scale 16: Fitness/Being in Shape

No.	Item	M	SD	$r_{(i;t-i)}$
53)	. . . I recovered well physically	3.28 **3.15**	1.13 **1.47**	.70 **.68**
61)	. . . I was in a good condition physically	3.26 **3.04**	1.09 **1.56**	.79 **.78**
69)	. . . I felt very energetic	2.91 **2.98**	1.15 **1.46**	.69 **.64**
75)	. . . my body felt strong	2.90 **2.94**	1.19 **1.53**	.79 **.82**

Scale 17: Burnout/Personal Accomplishment

No.	Item	M	SD	$r_{(i;t-i)}$
55)	. . . I accomplished many worthwhile things in my sport	2.94 **3.09**	1.23 **1.61**	.41 **.32**
60)	. . . I dealt very effectively with my teammates' problems	2.46 **2.94**	1.29 **1.81**	.65 **.64**
70)	. . . I easily understood how my teammates felt about things	3.11 **2.90**	1.32 **1.47**	.70 **.52**
77)	. . . I deal with emotional problems in my sport very calmly	2.72 **3.34**	1.24 **1.58**	.73 **.57**

Scale 18: Self-Efficacy

No.	Item	M	SD	$r_{(i;t-i)}$
52)	. . . I was convinced I could achieve my set goals during performance	3.34 **3.20**	1.28 **1.67**	.79 **.77**
	. . . I was convinced that I could achieve my performance at any time	3.20 **2.77**	1.34 **1.85**	.83 **.70**
65)	. . . I was convinced that I performed well	3.28 **3.07**	1.19 **1.57**	.78 **.78**
71)	. . . I was convinced that I had trained well	3.83 **3.49**	1.13 **1.64**	.68 **.74**

Scale 19: Self-Regulation

No.	Item	M	SD	$r_{(i;t-i)}$
56)	. . . I prepared myself mentally for performance	3.37 **3.01**	1.10 **1.56**	.63 **.65**
62)	. . . I pushed myself during performance	3.77 **3.84**	1.06 **1.54**	.65 **.56**
67)	. . . I psyched myself up before performance	3.32 **2.86**	1.19 **1.58**	.79 **.76**
74)	. . . I set definite goals for myself during performance	4.33 **3.17**	1.26 **1.62**	.57 **.68**

Brief Instructions for the RESTQ-Sport Database Program

The database program described in this manual offers computer support for analyzing data from both versions of the RESTQ-Sport questionnaire (52 or 76 items). Both versions have the same data input, profile calculation, and graphical presentation programming functions. The profile calculation offers the following options:

- Profile calculation for individuals and groups in a single trial
- Profile calculation for individuals and groups over multiple trials

The various functions of the RESTQ-Sport program are explained in more detail in the remainder of this document.

Let's begin with the system requirements and the installation instructions.

Minimum System Requirements

This CD-ROM can be installed on a Windows®-based PC.

- IBM PC compatible with Pentium® processor, or higher
- Windows® 9.x/NT 4.0 or Windows 2000
- At least 16 MB RAM with 32 MB recommended
- 2x CD-ROM drive
- 15 MB hard drive space available
- Inkjet or laser printer (optional)
- 256 colors
- VGA color monitor (800 × 600)
- Mouse

Windows® and Microsoft® are registered trademarks of Microsoft Corporation.

Installing the RESTQ-Sport Database Program

Microsoft Windows®

1. Close all current Windows applications.
2. Insert the *RESTQ-Sport CD-ROM* into the CD-ROM drive.
3. Select the Windows "Start" button.
4. Select the "Run…" option.
5. Type "X:\ RESTQ-Sport.exe" in the text box. (Note: X is the letter that corresponds to your CD-ROM drive.)
6. Follow the on-screen instructions to install the software.

Getting Started

Microsoft Windows®

1. Select the Windows "Start" button.
2. Select the "Programs" option.
3. Select the "RESTQ-Sport" program group.
4. Select the "RESTQ-Sport" icon.
5. Select the database you would like to work with. Restq.mdb is a sample database. To create your own, select Restq-master.mdb.

For product information or customer support:

E-mail: support@hkusa.com

Phone: 217-351-5076

Fax: 217-351-2674

Web site: **www.humankinetics.com**

The Program

The following is a general summary of the various programming areas and their functions.

At the start of the program, you will be asked to choose a database. To open a new database, choose "restq_master.mbd." The file restq.mdb is an example file to demonstrate how the database can be used when data are entered.

After starting up the program, the *Data Input* and *Graphical View* windows appear overlapped. Either window can be moved to the foreground by clicking on it, causing the other window to move to the background.

Data Input

In the data input window, data can be added or changed (figure B.1). **Some of the requested information is obligatory and some is optional.**

Single Code

Only one single code (personal code) with a maximum of 8 numbers or letters may be entered for each database because this code represents a particular individual. *The program's search mode cannot distin-* *guish between identical personal codes even if the group code is different.* **Obligatory input.**

If you have more than one team or group of athletes, a three-digit personal code may also be used. The first digit represents the team; the second and third digits represent the athlete. Examples: 101 (1: soccer; 01: athlete no.); 205 (2: handball; 05: athlete no.); 321 (3: basketball; 21: athlete no.). You can determine your own sport and team codes.

Group Code

A group code must also be entered. This code can consist of numbers or a combination of numbers and letters (with a maximum of 10 numbers or letters) and is used to specify the group for the analysis. In this case, the same code can be used that was chosen to specify the personal code (the first digit in the three-digit number). However, a letter code is recommended to have a better distinction between single and group codes. **Obligatory input.**

Last Name

Enter the last name of the individual. **Optional input.**

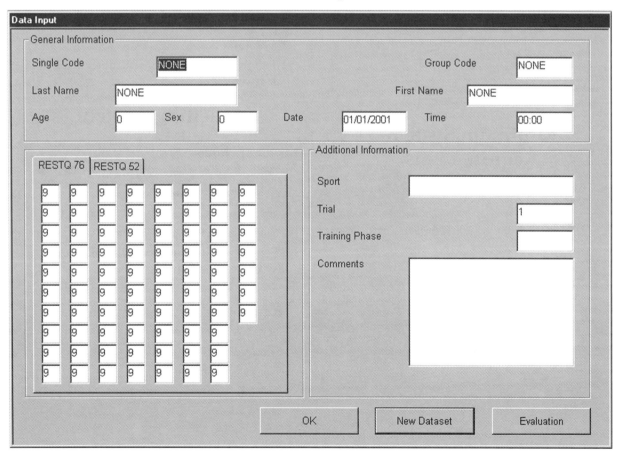

Figure B.1 Data input window.

First Name

Enter the first name of the individual. **Optional input.**

Age

Enter the age given on the questionnaire. **Obligatory input.**

Sex

Enter *0* for *female,* *1* for *male,* and *2* for *no information.* **Obligatory input.**

Date

The date must be an eight-digit number (mm/dd/yyyy). Check that the date is properly written. If it is not, you may not continue. **Obligatory input.**

Time

The same requirements apply for the time (mm:hh) as for the date. **Obligatory input.**

RESTQ-76/RESTQ-52 Buttons

Select the button that corresponds to the version of the questionnaire (RESTQ-76 or RESTQ-52) to be entered and start inputting the data. In case of missing data, enter the number 9. After entering the 9, use the mouse or the Tab key to move to the next input box and continue with inputting data.

Recommendation for the evaluation: If at least 50% of the information is completed in each scale, the program will substitute the missing data with a mean value from the existing items on that scale. The mean value for each item from the versions with 52 and 76 items will be used in calculating the results. **Obligatory input.**

Sport

Enter the name of the sport/event. **Optional input.**

Trial

This input provides information about which trial (i.e., "time of measurement") is being considered. This information is required for analyzing the data, especially if changes from one trial to the next are to be demonstrated. **Obligatory input.**

Training Phase

This input documents which training phase the athlete is in. Here you may develop your own scale schemata (i.e., weekly input during a one-year cycle). **Optional input.**

Comments

In this box, enter the current personal comments. **Optional input.**

OK Button

Click on this button to end the input for the current set of data and copy it into the database. You also can use this button to save changes which occur at a later date (e.g., adding/deleting comments, sport, or training phase).

New Dataset Button

Click on this button to save the previous dataset input and begin entering a new dataset.

Evaluation Button

Click on this button to bring up the dialog box for the profile calculation. While in the data setting, you may navigate by using the control panel (figure B.2) or menu entries.

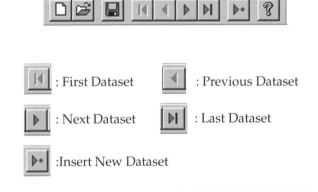

Figure B.2   Control panel functions.

Evaluation Function

Using data input or the upper symbol border, press *evaluation,* and a diagram will appear (figure B.3).

You must now choose to evaluate either an individual or a group (all athletes with the same group code).

Single Code Option

Select the single code for an individual and enter whether you want to compare the data from a single trial or—if available—from multiple trials.

If using a **single trial**, you have an additional option of defining the profile.

Without:

Profile without the "area of tolerance" (mean value ± one standard deviation)

Group:

Profile with reference to the "area of tolerance" at the same evaluation trial for the whole group

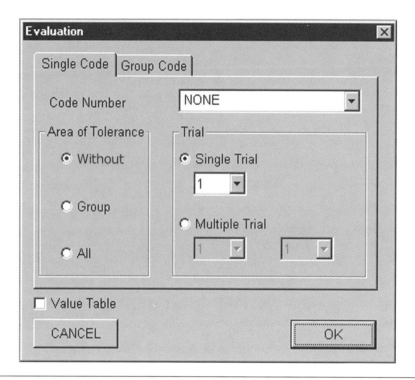

Figure B.3 The evaluation window.

All:

Profile with reference to the "area of tolerance" on all the available data settings in the database

Note: Calculation of the "area of tolerance" is only recommended for the whole group if at least eight individuals are considered at a given trial.

Using **multiple trials,** the profiles can only compare two different trials of one individual with each other. The number of profiles was limited so that the results can be clearly understood. This option also allows the comparison of nonconsecutive trials (3 vs. 9) in order to compare the development between different training phases. Only those profiles that refer to the same individual can be demonstrated. A direct comparison of different individuals is not possible.

Group Code Option

Select the group code and enter whether you want to compare the data from a single trial or—if available—from multiple trials.

If using a **single trial,** you have the option of defining the profile.

Without:

Profile without the "area of tolerance" (mean value ± one standard deviation)

All:

Profile with reference to the "area of tolerance" on all the available data settings in the database. This option is only meaningful for certain questions.

Using **multiple trials,** the profiles can only compare two different trials with each other. The number of profiles was limited so that the results can be clearly understood. Only those profiles that refer to the same group can be demonstrated. A direct comparison of different groups is not possible.

Value Table Option

Choosing this option brings up a value table of the selected trials, which appears on the right-hand side of the profile.

Profile Calculation Function

After determining the setup for the profile definition, enter OK. The window with the graphical presentation will appear in the foreground (figure B.4). To print this window, click on the print button.

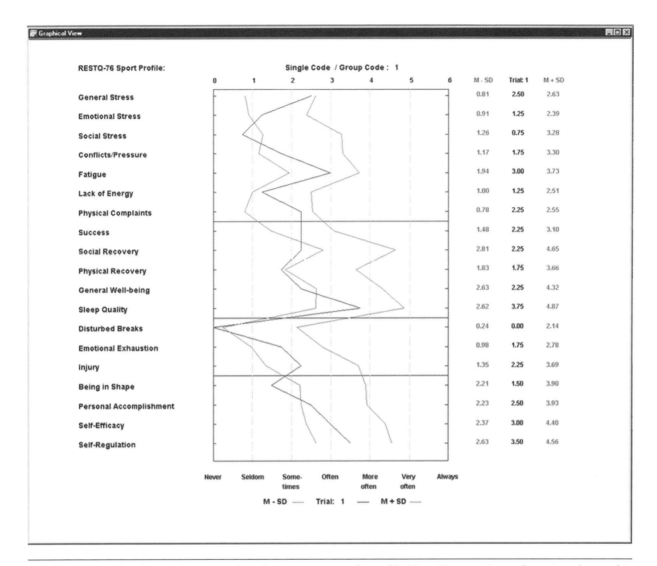

Figure B.4   Graphical presentation window showing an example profile. Note: Due to printer adaptation, the graphic printout may differ from one printer to another. In certain cases, we recommend changing the text to horizontal format.

Save the Database

Using the function "Save As" the restq_master.mdb can be saved under a different file name. The program does not allow to overwrite the file restq_master.mdb. *Note:* If you open the data file with Microsoft Access® and transfer the data into a statistics program, be aware that missing data are scored with a 9. Be sure not to modify the original data file because you may lose your data during the file conversion.

Feedback

To enhance the usability and productivity of the RESTQ-Sport, I would appreciate any feedback about your practical experience with the questionnaire and the data analysis. I would also be grateful if you would allow me access to your datasets for further analysis. Please send comments or data files via e-mail to the following address: **kellmann@rz.uni-potsdam.de**

R E S T Q - 52 Sport

Single Code:_____   Group Code:_____

Name (Last):_____   **(First):** _____

Age: _____   Gender: _____   Date: _____   Time: _____

Sport/Event(s): _____

This questionnaire consists of a series of statements. These statements possibly describe your psychic or physical well-being or your activities during the past few days and nights.

Please select the answer that most accurately reflects your thoughts and activities. Indicate how often each statement was right in your case in the past days.

The statements related to performance should refer to performance during competition as well as during practice.

For each statement there are seven possible answers.

Please make your selection by marking the number corresponding to the appropriate answer.

Example:

In the past (3) days/nights

... I read a newspaper

0	1	2	3	4	5	6
never	seldom	sometimes	often	more often	very often	always

In this example, the number 5 is marked. This means that you read a newspaper very often in the past three days.

Please do not leave any statements blank.

If you are unsure which answer to choose, select the one that most closely applies to you.

Please turn the page and respond to the statements in order without interruption.

From *Recovery-Stress Questionnaire for Athletes: User Manual* by Michael Kellmann and K. Wolfgang Kallus, 2001, Champaign, IL: Human Kinetics. **D.1**

In the past (3) days/nights

1) ... I watched TV

0	1	2	3	4	5	6
never	seldom	sometimes	often	more often	very often	always

2) ... I laughed

0	1	2	3	4	5	6
never	seldom	sometimes	often	more often	very often	always

3) ... I was in a bad mood

0	1	2	3	4	5	6
never	seldom	sometimes	often	more often	very often	always

4) ... I felt physically relaxed

0	1	2	3	4	5	6
never	seldom	sometimes	often	more often	very often	always

5) ... I was in good spirits

0	1	2	3	4	5	6
never	seldom	sometimes	often	more often	very often	always

6) ... I had difficulties in concentrating

0	1	2	3	4	5	6
never	seldom	sometimes	often	more often	very often	always

7) ... I worried about unresolved problems

0	1	2	3	4	5	6
never	seldom	sometimes	often	more often	very often	always

8) ... I had a god time with my friends

0	1	2	3	4	5	6
never	seldom	sometimes	often	more often	very often	always

9) ... I had a headache

0	1	2	3	4	5	6
never	seldom	sometimes	often	more often	very often	always

10) ... I was dead tired after work

0	1	2	3	4	5	6
never	seldom	sometimes	often	more often	very often	always

11) ... I was successful in what I did

0	1	2	3	4	5	6
never	seldom	sometimes	often	more often	very often	always

12) ... I felt uncomfortable

0	1	2	3	4	5	6
never	seldom	sometimes	often	more often	very often	always

D.2 From *Recovery-Stress Questionnaire for Athletes: User Manual* by Michael Kellmann and K. Wolfgang Kallus, 2001, Champaign, IL: Human Kinetics.

In the past (3) days/nights

13) ... I was annoyed by others

0	1	2	3	4	5	6
never	seldom	sometimes	often	more often	very often	always

14) ... I felt down

0	1	2	3	4	5	6
never	seldom	sometimes	often	more often	very often	always

15) ... I had a satisfying sleep

0	1	2	3	4	5	6
never	seldom	sometimes	often	more often	very often	always

16) ... I was fed up with everything

0	1	2	3	4	5	6
never	seldom	sometimes	often	more often	very often	always

17) ... I was in a good mood

0	1	2	3	4	5	6
never	seldom	sometimes	often	more often	very often	always

18) ... I was overtired

0	1	2	3	4	5	6
never	seldom	sometimes	often	more often	very often	always

19) ... I slept restlessly

0	1	2	3	4	5	6
never	seldom	sometimes	often	more often	very often	always

20) ... I was annoyed

0	1	2	3	4	5	6
never	seldom	sometimes	often	more often	very often	always

21) ... I felt as if I could get everything done

0	1	2	3	4	5	6
never	seldom	sometimes	often	more often	very often	always

22) ... I was upset

0	1	2	3	4	5	6
never	seldom	sometimes	often	more often	very often	always

23) ... I put off making decisions

0	1	2	3	4	5	6
never	seldom	sometimes	often	more often	very often	always

24) ... I made important decisions

0	1	2	3	4	5	6
never	seldom	sometimes	often	more often	very often	always

From *Recovery-Stress Questionnaire for Athletes: User Manual* by Michael Kellmann and K. Wolfgang Kallus, 2001, Champaign, IL: **D.3**
Human Kinetics.

In the past (3) days/nights

25) *... I felt under pressure*

0	1	2	3	4	5	6
never	seldom	sometimes	often	more often	very often	always

26) *... parts of my body were aching*

0	1	2	3	4	5	6
never	seldom	sometimes	often	more often	very often	always

27) *... I could not get rest during the breaks*

0	1	2	3	4	5	6
never	seldom	sometimes	often	more often	very often	always

28) *... I was convinced I could achieve my set goals during performance*

0	1	2	3	4	5	6
never	seldom	sometimes	often	more often	very often	always

29) *... I recovered well physically*

0	1	2	3	4	5	6
never	seldom	sometimes	often	more often	very often	always

30) *... I felt burned out by my sport*

0	1	2	3	4	5	6
never	seldom	sometimes	often	more often	very often	always

31) *... I accomplished many worthwhile things in my sport*

0	1	2	3	4	5	6
never	seldom	sometimes	often	more often	very often	always

32) *... I prepared myself mentally for performance*

0	1	2	3	4	5	6
never	seldom	sometimes	often	more often	very often	always

33) *... my muscles felt stiff or tense during performance*

0	1	2	3	4	5	6
never	seldom	sometimes	often	more often	very often	always

34) *... I had the impression there were too few breaks*

0	1	2	3	4	5	6
never	seldom	sometimes	often	more often	very often	always

35) *... I was convinced that I could achieve my performance at any time*

0	1	2	3	4	5	6
never	seldom	sometimes	often	more often	very often	always

36) *... I dealt very effectively with my teammates' problems*

0	1	2	3	4	5	6
never	seldom	sometimes	often	more often	very often	always

D.4 From *Recovery-Stress Questionnaire for Athletes: User Manual* by Michael Kellmann and K. Wolfgang Kallus, 2001, Champaign, IL: Human Kinetics.

In the past (3) days/nights

37) ... *I was in a good condition physically*

0	1	2	3	4	5	6
never	seldom	sometimes	often	more often	very often	always

38) ... *I pushed myself during performance*

0	1	2	3	4	5	6
never	seldom	sometimes	often	more often	very often	always

39) ... *I felt emotionally drained from performance*

0	1	2	3	4	5	6
never	seldom	sometimes	often	more often	very often	always

40) ... *I had muscle pain after performance*

0	1	2	3	4	5	6
never	seldom	sometimes	often	more often	very often	always

41) ... *I was convinced that I performed well*

0	1	2	3	4	5	6
never	seldom	sometimes	often	more often	very often	always

42) ... *too much was demanded of me during the breaks*

0	1	2	3	4	5	6
never	seldom	sometimes	often	more often	very often	always

43) ... *I psyched myself up before performance*

0	1	2	3	4	5	6
never	seldom	sometimes	often	more often	very often	always

44) ... *I felt that I wanted to quit my sport*

0	1	2	3	4	5	6
never	seldom	sometimes	often	more often	very often	always

45) ... *I felt very energetic*

0	1	2	3	4	5	6
never	seldom	sometimes	often	more often	very often	always

46) ... *I easily understood how my teammates felt about things*

0	1	2	3	4	5	6
never	seldom	sometimes	often	more often	very often	always

47) ... *I was convinced that I had trained well*

0	1	2	3	4	5	6
never	seldom	sometimes	often	more often	very often	always

48) ... *the breaks were not at the right times*

0	1	2	3	4	5	6
never	seldom	sometimes	often	more often	very often	always

From *Recovery-Stress Questionnaire for Athletes: User Manual* by Michael Kellmann and K. Wolfgang Kallus, 2001, Champaign, IL: **D.5**
Human Kinetics.

In the past (3) days/nights

49) ... I felt vulnerable to injuries

0	1	2	3	4	5	6
never	seldom	sometimes	often	more often	very often	always

50) ... I set definite goals for myself during performance

0	1	2	3	4	5	6
never	seldom	sometimes	often	more often	very often	always

51) ... my body felt strong

0	1	2	3	4	5	6
never	seldom	sometimes	often	more often	very often	always

52) ... I felt frustrated by my sport

0	1	2	3	4	5	6
never	seldom	sometimes	often	more often	very often	always

53) ... I dealt with emotional problems in my sport very calmly

0	1	2	3	4	5	6
never	seldom	sometimes	often	more often	very often	always

Thank you very much!

D.6 From *Recovery-Stress Questionnaire for Athletes: User Manual* by Michael Kellmann and K. Wolfgang Kallus, 2001, Champaign, IL: Human Kinetics.

Scales and Items of the RESTQ-52 Sport

Scale 1: General Stress
14) ... I felt down
16) ... I was fed up with everything

Scale 2: Emotional Stress
3) ... I was in a bad mood
20) ... I was annoyed

Scale 3: Social Stress
13) ... I was annoyed by others
22) ... I was upset

Scale 4: Conflicts/Pressure
7) ... I worried about unresolved problems
25) ... I felt under pressure

Scale 5: Fatigue
10) ... I was dead tired after work
18) ... I was overtired

Scale 6: Lack of Energy
6) ... I had difficulties in concentrating
23) ... I put off making decisions

Scale 7: Somatic Complaints
9) ... I had a headache
12) ... I felt uncomfortable

Scale 8: Success
11) ... I was successful in what I did
24) ... I made important decisions

Scale 9: Social Relaxation
2) ... I laughed
8) ... I had a good time with my friends

Scale 10: Somatic Relaxation
4) ... I felt physically relaxed
21) ... I felt as if I could get everything done

Scale 11: General Well-being
5) ... I was in good spirits
17) ... I was in a good mood

From *Recovery-Stress Questionnaire for Athletes: User Manual* by Michael Kellmann and K. Wolfgang Kallus, 2001, Champaign, IL: Human Kinetics.

Scale 12: Sleep Quality

15) ... I had a satisfying sleep
19) ... I slept restlessly

Scale 13: Disturbed Breaks

27) ... I could not get rest during the breaks
34) ... I had the impression there were too few breaks
42) ... too much was demanded of me during the breaks
48) ... the breaks were not at the right times

Scale 14: Burnout/Emotional Exhaustion

30) ... I felt burned out by my sport
39) ... I felt emotionally drained from performance
44) ... I felt that I wanted to quit my sport
52) ... I felt frustrated by my sport

Scale 15: Fitness/Injury

26) ... parts of my body were aching
33) ... my muscles felt stiff or tense during performance
40) ... I had muscle pain after performance
49) ... I felt vulnerable to injuries

Scale 16: Fitness/Being in Shape

29) ... I recovered well physically
37) ... I was in a good condition physically
45) ... I felt very energetic
51) ... my body felt strong

Scale 17: Burnout/Personal Accomplishment

31) ... I accomplished many worthwhile things in my sport
36) ... I dealt very effectively with my teammates' problems
46) ... I easily understood how my teammates felt about things
53) ... I dealt with emotional problems in my sport very calmly

Scale 18: Self-Efficacy

28) ... I was convinced I could achieve my set goals during performance
35) ... I was convinced that I could achieve my performance at any time
41) ... I was convinced that I performed well
47) ... I was convinced that I had trained well

Scale 19: Self-Regulation

32) ... I prepared myself mentally for performance
38) ... I pushed myself during performance
43) ... I psyched myelf up before performance
50) ... I set definite goals for myself during performance

Note: The item 19 of Sleep Quality has to be inverted for analysis.